Recommended by

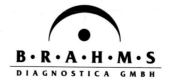

B·R·A·H·M·S
DIAGNOSTICA GMBH

Procalcitonin

A new, innovative infection parameter

Biochemical and clinical aspects

Dr. med. Michael Meisner

3rd revised and extended edition
57 figures, 23 tables

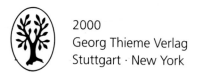

2000
Georg Thieme Verlag
Stuttgart · New York

Dr. med. Michael Meisner
Friedrich-Schiller-University of Jena
Department of Anaesthesiology and
Intensive Care Therapy
Bachstr. 18
07743 Jena
Germany

Die Deutsche Bibliothek – CIP-Einheitsaufnahme

Meisner, Michael:
Procalcitonin : a new, innovative infection parameter ; biochemical and clinical aspects ; 23
tables / Michael Meisner. – 3., rev. and expanded
ed.. – Stuttgart ; New York : Thieme, 2000
    Dt. Ausg. u.d.T.: Meisner, Michael: Procalci-
tonin

1st and 2nd edition published by
Fa. B·R·A·H·M·S Diagnostica GmbH

© 2000 Georg Thieme Verlag
Rüdigerstraße 14
D-70469 Stuttgart

Printed in Germany

Printing: Druckhaus Götz GmbH, Ludwigsburg
Bookbinding: F. W. Held, Rottenburg

ISBN 3-13-105503-0   4 5 6

Preface to the 3rd Edition

Our knowledge about PCT has rapidly expanded over the last two years and many new publications on the subject of PCT have come to light. We therefore need to review the results obtained to date and to make the information available to the interested reader in a completely revised edition of the monograph.

PCT is increasingly recognized as an important diagnostic tool in clinical practice. PCT is far more suitable for detecting complications of bacterial infection characterized by systemic inflammatory reactions than other parameters. High plasma levels are observed in situations characterized by the onset of organ dysfunction or the symptoms of "severe sepsis" or "septic shock". These are clinically relevant conditions warranting various intensive therapeutic interventions. The extent to which PCT is triggered by non-bacterial infections has also been reported in various publications. PCT levels may rise following major surgery or in multiple trauma patients but are less marked than in cases of sepsis or septic shock. These observations do not, however, limit the diagnostic benefits of PCT. On the contrary, PCT serves to identify risk groups following major surgery or in multiple trauma patients. There are obviously diagnostic limitations with this parameter, especially in cases where only a small quantity of PCT is induced and simultaneous induction occurs due to trauma. Particular attention will be devoted to this subject in the monograph.

The origin of inflammatory-induced PCT has not been fully elucidated. There is, however, evidence to suggest that macrophage and monocyte system cells are capable of synthesising PCT. The fact that bacterial endotoxins are a strong inducer of PCT as well as the fact that individual pro-inflammatory cytokines are also capable of PCT induction has been confirmed in tests conducted in model systems.

The attentive reader may also inquire why numerous short publications and abstracts are quoted in this book. Developments in the area of PCT are so rapid that exclusion of this reference material would result in information being withheld from the reader. The aim of this monograph is nevertheless to make available expert information which cannot be found in any data network and which the interested reader would find time-consuming to review if he/she had access to it in the first place.

Finally, up-to-the-minute information and data on PCT are available on the Internet. Visit the website at **http://www.procalci tonin.com** for access to numerous data banks and information on PCT. This includes an open forum for discussion regarding clinical studies, assess specific queries and to promote contact between experts and users.

I am indebted to **B·R·A·H·M·S Diagnostica GmbH**, Hennigsdorf/Berlin, for giving me the opportunity to produce and publish this monograph. I am especially grateful to all the authors and research groups who provided me with rapid, straightforward information and data for inclusion in this work.

At this point, I would also like to thank the many scientists, clinicians, colleagues and PhD students investigating the topic of PCT who have contributed to the latest findings in this interesting field of research. Users should not hesitate to contact the author or colleagues working in individual research groups if they have any specific questions on PCT or wish to plan and discuss additional projects and studies.

Jena, April 2000

Dr. med. Michael Meisner

1 Introduction

1.1 Procalcitonin (PCT)

Numerous laboratory parameters are currently available for the diagnosis of inflammatory diseases and characterization of the immune response. Specific laboratory tests accurately identify the type and activity of on-going inflammation. In daily routine diagnosis, however, there are few parameters available to monitor critically ill patients and to monitor the course of therapy in severe inflammatory conditions. There are also few reliable parameters with clinical utility in the differential diagnosis of inflammatory conditions and the resulting clinical assessment is often uncertain. With the launch of procalcitonin (PCT) in 1996, a diagnostic tool became available for identifying severe bacterial infections and reliably indicating complications secondary to systemic inflammation. PCT levels increase in cases of sepsis, septic shock and in severe systemic inflammatory reactions. Compared to other parameters, PCT facilitates reliable follow-up of the clinical course of these conditions.

The main stimulus for PCT induction under experimental conditions is the systemic effect of bacterial endotoxins (LPS). Viral diseases, autoimmune diseases, neoplastic disorders and local and organ-related bacterial infections do not induce PCT. PCT can therefore be used for the differential diagnosis of bacterial and non-bacterial disorders. Moreover, PCT can also be used to monitor patients at risk of infection or sepsis for the early detection of infectious complications. This application is particularly important in high-risk surgical and immunosuppressed patients. PCT is also frequently induced in systemic fungal infections accompanied by a severe systemic inflammatory reaction.

With an *in-vivo* half-life of 20–24 hours and high stability in serum or plasma *ex-vivo*, PCT possesses ideal criteria for a daily parameter. A once-daily determination is generally adequate for the diagnosis and monitoring of septic patients and patients at risk for developing septic complications. PCT can be determined in the laboratory with LUMItest® PCT or at the point of care for rapid differential diagnosis. The semi-quantitative rapid test now available (B·R·A·H·M·S PCT®-Q) will greatly facilitate this type of use in the future.

The biochemical properties of PCT, its induction mechanisms and potential functions in immune reactions are discussed in the following chapters. The role of PCT in monitoring therapeutic intervention and for assessing the prognosis of septic patients is discussed in a separate chapter. Special indications for the determination of PCT in the differential diagnosis of bacterial and non-bacterial diseases are discussed in Chapter 4. The course of PCT is also compared with other inflammatory parameters using case report examples. The technical aspects of the PCT measuring kits produced by B·R·A·H·M·S Diagnostica GmbH, Hennigsdorf/Berlin are discussed in Chapters 5 and 6.

The purpose of this monograph is to publish the experience with PCT to date in summary format in order to highlight the potential benefit and limitations of infection diagnosis using this new parameter.

1.2   Indications for the determination of PCT

PCT (procalcitonin) is indicated for use primarily as a diagnostic parameter for bacterial infections triggering a systemic-inflammatory reaction in the body (sepsis, septic shock). Local limited bacterial or organ-related infections and capsulated abscesses induce a slight increase in PCT if at all. Immunosuppression and neutropenia do not significantly affect PCT formation. Bacterial toxins play a crucial role in the induction of PCT. Diseases, the etiology and course of which involve bacterial endotoxins, such as sepsis, septic shock, systemic inflammation and multiple organ dysfunction syndrome (MODS) are characterized by very high PCT concentrations often ranging from 10 to 100 ng/ml and up to 1,000 ng/ml in certain individual cases. Non-specific, *i.e.* infection-independent induction of PCT, may occur after major surgery, multiple trauma or in newborn infants during the first days of life. In these instances, values rarely exceed 5 ng/ml.

PCT induction and the increase in plasma levels are closely correlated with the extent and type of systemic inflammation. Both the underlying disease and the anatomical extent of the infected tissue play a role. Once the acute inflammation has waned, PCT concentrations rapidly fall. PCT can be used to monitor therapy after surgical removal of a bacterial focus. Also in the course of septic diseases, PCT reflects the severity of the disease and the course of the inflammatory activity. Hence PCT is not only a monitoring marker in the course of sepsis, but also a marker for the prognosis and success of therapeutic procedures. Elevated PCT plasma levels correlate with the course of severe septic diseases characterized by arterial hypotension and impaired organ perfusion. PCT is therefore also an indicator of the severity of systemic inflammation secondary to infection.

Because of these pathophysiological properties, PCT can be used for the differential diagnosis of the etiology of acute inflammation. It can also be used as a marker with a broad range of infectious indications and for monitoring patients at risk of sepsis or who are critically ill.

1.3　　A survey of primary indications

The primary indications for use and key applications of PCT known to date are discussed in this survey. The indications for use are categorized into five groups:

Diagnosis of infection with systemic inflammation

In healthy people, PCT plasma concentrations are usually below the detection limit of the immunoluminometric assay. PCT concentrations above 0.5 ng/ml generally indicate an acute infection accompanied by a systemic inflammatory reaction. Particularly high PCT values have been reported in patients with severe bacterial infections and septic inflammation, *e.g.* severe sepsis or septic shock according to ACCP/SCCM criteria (5). Locally confined inflammatory reactions and infections or superficial bacterial colonization do not induce PCT or are associated only with moderately elevated PCT plasma concentrations.

Monitoring therapy and the course of bacterial infections

Serial measurement of PCT levels can be used to monitor the course of disease and to follow up a therapeutic regimen in all severe and potentially life-threatening bacterial infections, *e.g.* peritonitis, extended soft tissue infections or anastomotic leakage. Increasing PCT concentrations are an indication of generalized inflammation such as sepsis or the onset of septic shock. Decreasing PCT values usually indicate successful surgical removal of an inflammatory focus or adequate antibiotic therapy.

- Increasing PCT values or values which remain consistently high indicate continuing disease activity.
- A fall in PCT levels suggests waning of the inflammatory reaction and resolution of the infection.

Differential diagnosis of inflammatory diseases and fever of unknown origin

Beneficial experience with PCT is reported in the differential diagnosis of the following diseases:
- Differential diagnosis of sterile and infected necroses in acute pancreatitis
- Biliary versus toxic etiology of acute pancreatitis
- Bacterial versus viral meningitis in newborn infants and children
- Bacterial or non-infectious etiology of ARDS (acute respiratory distress syndrome)
- Differential diagnosis of infectious microbial-induced fever versus non-bacterial fever, *e.g.* in immunosuppressed patients
- Differential diagnosis of acute organ rejection versus post-transplantation infection
- Evidence of bacterial infections in autoimmune disorders with symptoms of acute inflammation

Diagnostic utility in the management of inflammatory diseases of unknown origin

The monitoring and management of critically ill patients
- routinely after major surgery
- monitoring of infection in patients with multiple trauma
- monitoring of infection following organ transplantation
- patients with a prolonged stay in the ICU (intensive care unit) and prolonged mechanical ventilation

Prognostic information and clinical management in sepsis, septic shock and multiple organ dysfunction syndrome (MODS)

- As a parameter for monitoring the course of sepsis and multiple organ dysfunction syndrome, PCT indicates the extent of the systemic inflammatory reaction.
- Increasing or persistent PCT values indicate poor patient prognosis.
- Declining PCT values suggest that the infection or inflammation is under control and indicate a good prognosis.

Additional diagnostic procedures can be implemented, or a treatment regimen changed or confirmed based on increasing or declining PCT values.

PCT in different medical fields

Numerous clinical studies have established the benefit of PCT in diagnosis and therapeutic management in different medical specialties. PCT provides additional information regarding the differential diagnosis and control of infection and severe inflammation compared with presently used and generally conducted diagnostic procedures, as indicated by the following examples:

Internal medicine

- for the early, reliable detection of septic diseases and rapid assessment of the degree of severity
- in acute pancreatitis for the differential diagnosis of infected versus sterile necroses and the early identification of biliary pancreatitis versus toxic etiologies
- for the identification of infectious etiologies in fever of unknown origin (FUO)
- for the differentiation of viral infections or acute exacerbation of an autoimmune disease versus acute bacterial infections in patients receiving immunosuppressive agents
- in ARDS for the differentiation between infectious versus non-infectious etiology

Hematology and oncology

- monitoring of immunosuppressed patients
- monitoring of neutropenic patients following chemotherapy
- differential diagnosis of fever induced by tumour lysis or chemotherapy in oncology patients versus infection-induced etiologies
- differentiation between viral and bacterial infections

Transplantation medicine

- differentiation between an acute organ rejection or viral infection versus bacterial infection
- as a general monitoring parameter for bacterial infections and to rule out systemic bacterial infection (sepsis)
- before transplantation to rule out acute bacterial infections

Pediatrics

- to aid the differential diagnosis of acute meningitis by differentiating between bacterial and viral etiologies
- in acute fever of neonates and infants for the diagnosis of systemic bacterial infection and the onset of sepsis versus non-septic diseases

Surgery and in the ICU

- in the post-operative period as an early indicator of bacterial and septic infectious complications
- for the management of successful therapy after surgical elimination of infectious foci (peritonitis, soft tissue infections)
- for monitoring the course of disease in peritonitis, anastomotic leakage and non-specific abdominal symptoms
- for the rapid diagnosis of sepsis
- for monitoring patients at risk of sepsis
- for monitoring the course of a disease and therapeutic management in patients presenting with systemic inflammation and sepsis

2 Biochemistry

2.1 Biosynthesis and peptide structure

Procalcitonin (PCT) is a 116 amino acid protein with a sequence identical to that of the prohormone of calcitonin (32 amino acids) (Figure 2.1.1) (91, 136). Under normal metabolic conditions, hormonally active calcitonin is produced and secreted in the C-cells of the thyroid gland after specific intracellular proteolytic procession of the prohormone procalcitonin. In severe bacterial infections and sepsis, however, intact procalcitonin is found in blood. Current research indicates that the orgin of procalcitonin in these conditions is extrathyroidal.

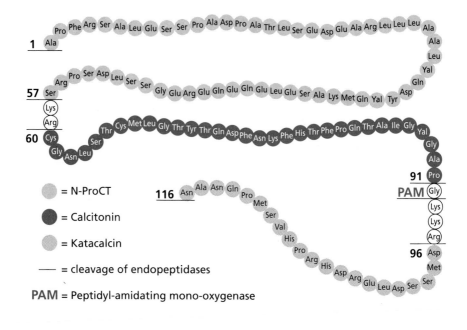

Figure 2.1.1

Schematic description of the aminoacid sequence of PCT (according to 91).

Normal values and reference ranges

Plasma concentrations of the prohormone procalcitonin in healthy individuals are substantially below 0.1 ng/ml and thus below the detection limit of the LUMItest® PCT assay. In severe bacterial infections, however, high plasma concentrations of PCT are found without any significant change in calcitonin levels. Plasma PCT is very stable and is not degraded to hormonally active calcitonin. In cases of severe sepsis, concentrations of PCT ranging from below 10 ng/ml to over 1000 ng/ml are found in plasma. The reference ranges are listed on page 175.

Procalcitonin, fragments thereof and other precursor peptides of calcitonin can be detected in small quantities (picogram per millilitre range) in the plasma of healthy subjects (18, 153, 166). Accurate measurement of PCT concentrations below 0.5 ng/ml will be possible in the future using ultrasensitive measuring techniques. PCT induction may also be detected in localized or systemically inactive infections using ultrasensitive techniques. The normal range for procalcitonin in the LUMItest® PCT assay is currently given as <0.5 ng/ml PCT based on PCT concentrations in a large normal patient population.

PCT synthesis

C-cells of the thyroid are not believed to be the source of bacterial infection induced PCT. Other cells including macrophages and monocytic cells of various organs, e.g. the liver, are believed to be involved in the synthesis and release of PCT in response to bacterial infections. It has been known for some time that synthesis of calcitonin precursor mRNA takes place in the liver (29).

Calcitonin and its precursor peptides are synthesized by leukocytes (129, 130) and neurocrine cells of internal organs such as the lung and the intestine (11, 19, 120, 160) as well as other cell types. In fact, using in-situ hybridization, induced mRNA production was recently detected in other cell types using the hamster as a model (179). Katacalcin and calcitonin were detected intracellularly in various types of human leukocytes by means of flow-cytometric analysis (FACS) (Figure 2.1.2) (130). Induced PCT mRNA was also observed in human monocytic blood cells via semi-quantitative polymerase chain reaction (PCR) using the reverse transcriptase technique (RT-PCR) (Figure 2.4.3.) (129, 130). It has not yet been confirmed whether the quantities of PCT released by these cells are adequate to account for the levels of PCT observed in septic patients (94, 171).

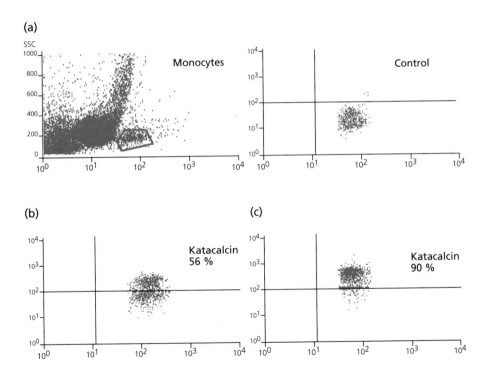

Figure 2.1.2 a-c

Detection by means of flow-through cytometric analysis of an intracellular katacalcin antibody reaction in patients with normal (b) and elevated (c) serum PCT values in a CD14-positive monocyte population. (a) Comparison of study population versus control (130).

In addition to PCT, other cleavage products of the calcitonin prohormone are found in plasma. However, PCT represents the main product of the calcitonin precursor peptides (18, 19, 119, 153, 166).

Elimination of PCT

A specific route of elimination for PCT has not been established. Like other plasma proteins, PCT is probably degraded by proteolysis. Renal excretion of PCT plays a minor role. Clinical data have shown that PCT does not accumulate in cases of severe renal dysfunction. The fall in plasma PCT concentrations observed in patients with renal dysfunction does not differ significantly from that of subjects with normal renal function (101, 172). In our own investigations, approximately one-quarter of the concentrations measured in plasma were detected in urine although the concentrations measured in urine fluctuated considerably. The renal clearance of plasma PCT was calculated to be markedly less than 1 ml/min (172). PCT could also be detected in the ultrafiltrate with continuous veno-venous hemofiltration (CVVHF) or in the dialysate with continuous hemodiafiltration (CVVHDF) (173, 174). A sieving coefficient of 0.24 was recorded for PCT. PCT clearance in plasma and ultrafiltrate ranged from 2 to over 5 ml/min in these studies. Filter adsorption phenomena were observed only during the first hour following the onset of artificial renal replacement therapy. PCT plasma concentrations were not significantly affected even during 24-hour hemofiltration or hemodiafiltration (173, 174). The determination of PCT can therefore be used for diagnostic purposes in patients presenting with renal failure or those receiving artificial renal replacement therapy.

The effect of PCT on calcium and phosphate concentrations

Evidence changes in serum calcium and phosphate levels were observed in only a few individual studies in patients with elevated PCT concentrations.

Slightly decreased calcium levels and elevated phosphate levels were reported by Nylen et al. (120) in patients with pneumonia.

No correlation between serum calcium and PCT could be established in studies conducted in malaria patients (47). Laboratory animal studies in the hamster confirmed a significant fall in serum calcium levels and an increase in serum phosphate concentrations with simultaneous elevation of plasma levels of calcitonin precursor proteins (including PCT) in a model of E. coli peritonitis (159). The role of PCT and other calcitonin precursor molecules in these changes has not been elucidated. Similarly, the physiological relevance of these observations has not been confirmed.

Synthesis of PCT and calcitonin

Synthesis of the proteins PCT and calcitonin is complex and starts with the translation of a 141 amino acid (AA) precursor peptide (preprocalcitonin). By specific intracellular proteolysis, initially procalcitonin (116 amino acids), then calcitonin (32 amino acids) are liberated from this peptide.

The processing and proteolytic cleavage of the peptides, including their precise peptide sequence, are discussed in the following chapter.

The interesting genomic regulation of the calcitonin gene and its transcription to preprocalcitonin is described in chapter 2.2.

The "Pre-pro-hormone"
After transcription of the CALC-1 gene, the primary transcript is processed into mRNA encoding a 141-amino acid protein with a molecular weight of approximately 16 kDa. This "precursor protein", preprocalcitonin, comprises a signal sequence, the N-terminal region of procalcitonin (N-PCT), the middle sequence of calcitonin and the C-terminal region of procalcitonin called "katacalcin" (Figure 2.1.3) (136).

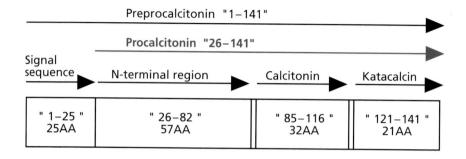

Figure 2.1.3

Preprocalcitonin, PCT and fragments (according to 136).

PCT, a glycoprotein?

The signal or leader sequence is a markedly hydrophobic sequence and mediates binding of the protein to the endoplasmic reticulum (ER). The ER is the most important structure of the cell for processing exocrine peptides. The signal sequence (AA 1-25) is degraded immediately after location in the ER by an endopeptidase, EP (Figure 2.1.4) (136), (Figure 2.1.5) (120). Precursor proteins of calcitonin can be glycosylated and are more stable against enzymatic degradation as glycoproteins than as asialoprotein (80). However, according to present knowledge, inflammatory-induced plasma PCT is not glycosylated.

Specific proteolysis

The resulting protein comprises 116 amino acids and is known as procalcitonin (PCT, Figure 2.1.1) (136). Within this polypeptide, the amino acid sequence of calcitonin can be found at position 60 to 91. This sequence is flanked by polybasic amino acids (Lys-Arg and Gly-Lys-Lys-Arg). These sequences are signal sequences for specific proteolysis by the enzyme prohormone convertase (PC), resulting in the main cleavage products of procalcitonin: N-PCT (57 AA), calcitonin (32 AA) and katacalcin (21 AA) and their combinations. This cleavage does not occur with inflammatory-induced PCT so that intact PCT can be found in plasma. It is interesting to note that amino acid sequences suitable for specific phosphorylation appear in the region between these cleavage products. The potential for inflammation-activated phosphorylation of PCT may be responsible for the presence of intact PCT in the plasma during sepsis and infection. Recent studies have shown that the amino acid chain of PCT N-terminal can be truncated by two amino acids

PREPROCALCITONIN

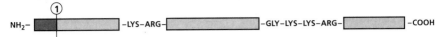

1. Cleavage of the signal peptide: ①

2. Glycosylation of asparagine 3 (hypothetical): ②

PROCALCITONIN

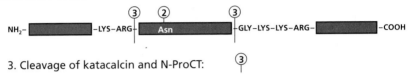

3. Cleavage of katacalcin and N-ProCT: ③

4. Cyclic formation by disulphide bridges:

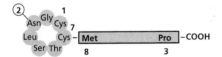

5. Amidation of proline 32

6. Deglycosylation of asparagine 3

CALCITONIN

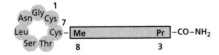

Figure 2.1.4

Biosynthesis of calcitonin via procalcitonin (according to 136).

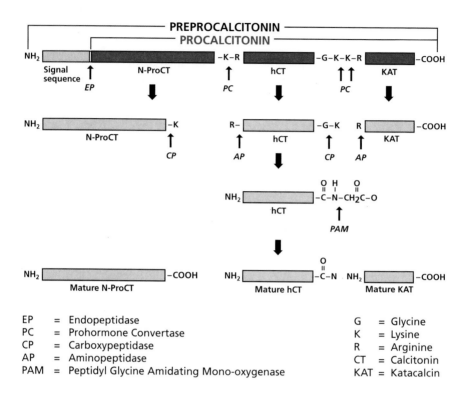

EP   = Endopeptidase
PC   = Prohormone Convertase
CP   = Carboxypeptidase
AP   = Aminopeptidase
PAM = Peptidyl Glycine Amidating Mono-oxygenase

G   = Glycine
K   = Lysine
R   = Arginine
CT   = Calcitonin
KAT = Katacalcin

Figure 2.1.5

Cleavage of preprocalcitonin by specific endopeptidases (according to 120).

(PCT 3-116) by the enzyme dipeptidyl peptidase IV (182). This does not, however, affect the measurements recorded with the LUMItest® PCT and B·R·A·H·M·S PCT®-Q.

The hormone calcitonin

The hormone calcitonin does not take on its final form until immediately after this cleavage process via cyclic formation of disulphide bridges (CysCys), cleavage of the C-terminal glycine (AS 3, carboxypeptidase) and subsequent amidation (peptidyl glycine amidating mono-oxygenase PAM) (Figure 2.1.5) (136). The hormone calcitonin is released into the circulating blood in healthy subjects. Calcitonin has a half-life of only a few minutes in blood (6).

Sepsis: calcitonin precursor molecules in plasma

With systemic inflammation secondary to severe bacterial infections, sepsis, septic shock and multiple organ dysfunction syndrome, high concentrations of stable calcitonin precursor peptides are found in the blood without corresponding calcitonin secretion (166). PCT is one of the principal precursor peptides and has a half-life of approximately 20 to 24 hours in plasma (101, 172).

Minor proteolysis in the plasma

It has been proposed that the targeted proteolytic cleavage of PCT in the Golgi apparatus is suppressed by the actions of cytokines and endotoxins so that the unprocessed precursor proteins including procalcitonin and its fragments are released into the circulating plasma (15, 166). At the same time, transcription of PCT mRNA is substantially increased by inflammatory stimuli (129). Unlike calcitonin, PCT is highly stable in plasma.

The appearance of high concentrations in the plasma can be attributed to the induction mechanisms described and the considerable stability of PCT.

The gene family of calcitonins

At present, four genes with nucleotide sequence homologies corresponding to calcitonin are known. These genes are collectively called the "calcitonin gene family", but they do not all produce the peptide hormone calcitonin. The "CALC-1" gene is responsible for the production of calcitonin and its precursor protein, procalcitonin. This gene may be responsible for the generation of inflammatory induced PCT.

The calcitonin gene (CALC-I) exhibits one of the first examples of a process termed alternative splicing. The primary RNA transcript is processed into different mRNA segments by inclusion or exclusion of different exons as part of the primary transcript. Calcitonin-encoding mRNA is the main product of CALC-I transcription in C-cells of the thyroid, whereas CGRP-I mRNA (CGRP = calcitonin-gene-related peptide) is produced in nervous tissue of the central and peripheral nervous systems (Figure 2.2.1) (9).

A computer-aided analysis of the sequence of the CALC-I gene promoter region known to date shows that, at least theoretically, different transcription factors activated by inflammation bind in this region and may influence transcription. Reporter gene construction could help to clarify the inflammatory-activated induction of PCT.

The primary transcript of the CALC-I gene produces 5 exons which can be combined to form three different mRNAs after transcription, maturation, splicing and polyadenylation. The resulting mRNA CT-1 and CT-2 encode pre-procalcitonin and differ only in the sequence of the carboxyterminal peptide I and II (Figure 2.2.1). In the third mRNA sequence, the calcitonin sequence is lost and alternatively the sequence of CGRP is encoded in the mRNA. CGRP is a markedly vasoactive peptide with vasodilatative properties. CGRP has no effect on calcium and phosphate metabolism (30) and is synthesised predominantly in nerve cells related to smooth muscle cells of the blood vessels (149). ProCGRP and PCT have partly identical N-terminal amino acid sequences.

Additional post-transcriptional processing can occur so that PCT is expressed with additional mRNA products (29, 168) and their corresponding translation products.

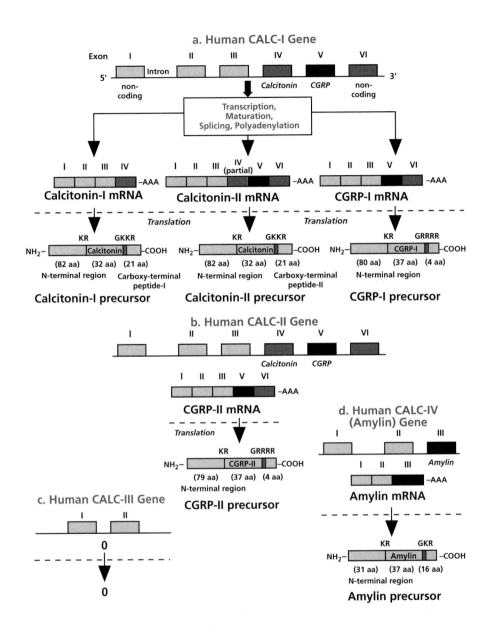

Figure 2.2.1

The human calcitonin gene family (according to 17).

The other genes do not contribute to calcitonin synthesis. The CALC-II gene has a similar structure to that of the CALC-I gene. Sequence analysis however indicates that the synthesis of calcitonin mRNA is unlikely. The CALC-II gene codes only for a CGRP-II precursor. CGRP-II differs from CGRP-I in 3 amino acids. The CALC-III gene is probably a pseudogene and does not transcribe any protein. The CALC-IV gene contains only 3 exons and codes for the amylin gene. This peptide has 46% sequence homology with the CGRP peptide. Amylin is a functional opponent of insulin (44).

Purely hypothetically, the occurrence of another gene of the calcitonin family is feasible, since production of inflammatory induced PCT obviously does not originate in the C-cells of the thyroid and, moreover, the regulation of the transcription of this gene is very similar to proinflammatory cytokines, particularly TNF-α and IL-6 (127). The detection of inducible PCT-mRNA via RT-PCR (129), inflammatory inducible induction of CGRP (82) and a computer-aided analysis of the promoter region of the CALC-I gene, which cannot rule out induction secondary to inflammation, nevertheless confirm that this is hypothetical.

Structural similarities in the organization of these genes may suggest that calcitonin and CGRP exons are derived from a primordial gene. The different genes and proteins of the calcitonin gene family may have arisen by gene duplication and events leading to sequence divergence (9, 17).

2.3 Systemic inflammation secondary to bacterial infection as the primary inducer of PCT

Elevated PCT levels indicate bacterial infection accompanied by a systemic inflammatory reaction. PCT production can be induced by bacterial endotoxins, exotoxins and certain cytokines. Increased plasma PCT concentrations are therefore detected in sepsis, septic shock as well as in systemic inflammation of varying etiologies such as multiple organ dysfunction syndrome (MODS). Elevated PCT levels have also been reported in patients presenting with malaria and in numerous cases of systemic fungal infection (4, 47, 64, 78).

PCT is slightly increased, if at all, in response to viral infections, neoplastic and autoimmune disorders. Chronic, non-bacterial inflammation and allergic reactions do not induce PCT.

Localized infections generally fail to trigger significant plasma PCT increases.

Normal plasma and serum concentrations of PCT are below 0.5 ng/ml. All values in excess of 0.5 ng/ml are considered abnormal. The range between 0.5 ng/ml to about 2 ng/ml is usually slightly elevated. Values of approximately 2 ng/ml to 5 ng/ml are considered moderately high whereas those exceeding 5 ng/ml are considered to be very high PCT values. According to many authors, PCT values in excess of 10 ng/ml are almost exclusively indicative of severe sepsis or septic shock.

Slightly elevated PCT concentrations (0.5 to 2.0 ng/ml) are observed in bacterial infections which have triggered a minor systemic inflammatory response. This range is especially important for differential diagnosis in acute diseases.

Very high values of over 10 ng/ml have been observed during acute disease conditions with severe systemic reactions to an infection, in cases of severe sepsis or septic shock and in MODS with underlying infection or sepsis. There have been isolated reports of plasma concentrations of over 1,000 ng/ml PCT.

Slightly increased PCT values have been observed in ICU patients or following surgery without any evidence of infection. Monitoring PCT levels has value in these patients. Due to the half-life of procalcitonin, a once-daily determination facilitates timely detection of any new infections or complications that may arise.

Familiarity with the expected range of plasma PCT concentrations in various patient groups or in disease states is essential for correct interpretation of PCT levels. This applies in particular to the post-surgical period (chapter 4.2), in multiple trauma patients (chapter 4.4), in patients presenting with extensive burns (chapter 4.15) and in newborn infants (chapter 4.16).

The level of PCT concentration is closely correlated with the type, extent and spread of the infection and, in particular, with the systemic manifestations of the inflammatory reaction. Bacterial infections which are confined to a single organ or which are not accompanied by symptoms of sepsis typically present with PCT levels that are not significantly raised. This is often the case with pneumonia in which the measured values are generally below 2 ng/ml. With the exception of protozoal (malaria) or fungal infections elevated levels rarely occur with non-bacterial diseases. This is also the case in very severe viral infections, autoimmune disorders, or neoplastic diseases (50, 75) in which values in excess of 2 ng/ml are rarely observed.

2.4 Induction mechanisms

The injection of bacterial endotoxin in healthy subjects

PCT synthesis can be stimulated in healthy subjects by injecting small quantities of bacterial endotoxins. PCT is initially detected in the plasma approximately 2–3 hours post-injection. Levels then rise rapidly, reaching a plateau after 6–12 hours. PCT concentrations remain high for up to 48 hours (46, 85, 136, 137), falling to their baseline values within the following 2 days (Figures 2.4.1 and 2.6.1) (46). The half-life is about 20 to 24 hours (40, 46, 101, 126, 172).

Case report: Accidental administration of a bacterially contaminated infusion solution

Brunkhorst et al. (40) reported on the administration of an accidentally contaminated infusion solution (contaminated with *Acinetobacter baumanii*) to a 76 year-old female patient who presented with dizziness, tachycardia and myalgia immediately after administration. The patient had a temperature of 40.3°C within 3 hours of administration; disseminated intravascular coagulation (DIC) developed after 9 hours. PCT levels were detected 3 hours post-administration with peak concentrations being reached after 14 hours (Figure 2.4.2). The half-life was 22.5 hours. C-reactive protein (CRP) levels were slightly increased after 12 hours, reaching a peak after 30 hours.

In-vitro models of PCT induction

Detection of PCT mRNA by means of RT-PCR facilitates investigation of the induction of PCT in cell cultures or blood cells (129). Bacterial endotoxins (lipopolysaccharides, LPS) are the most potent stimulators of PCT in these *in-vitro* studies. LPS triggers a 4-fold to 230-fold increase in PCT mRNA in peripheral blood mononuclear cells compared with unstimulated controls. In descending order, TNF-α, IL-6, IL-1β, IL-2 and phythohemagglutinin (PHA) also induce the production of PCT mRNA in these cells.

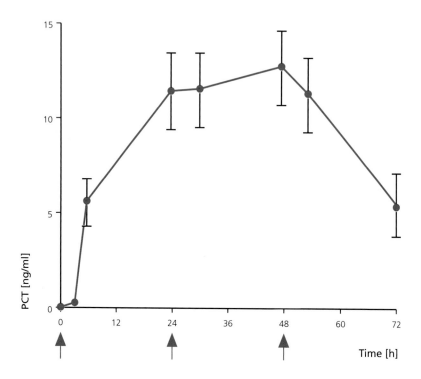

Figure 2.4.1

The plasma PCT concentrations (ng/ml) of 5 patients after 3 repeated endotoxin injections (*Salmonella abortus* equi. 4 ng/kg body weight at times 0h, 24h and 48h). The results are expressed as the mean value ± standard deviation from the mean (SEM) (according to 46).

No induction was observed with IL-10 (Figure 2.4.3) (129). Whereas a transient rise in intracellular concentrations can be observed following protein stimulation, no significant release of PCT into the culture medium occurred following incubation with LPS both in whole blood and in isolates of peripheral monocytic cells (94). It cannot be confirmed at the present time whether this was due to an inadequate stimulus or whether PCT actually originates from another source.

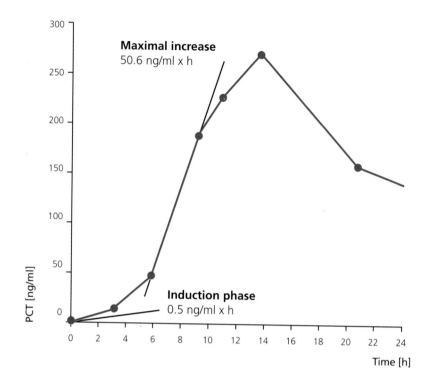

Figure 2.4.2

PCT plasma concentrations (ng/ml) following infusion of an accidentally bacterially (*Acinetobacter baumanii*) contaminated infusion solution to a 76 year-old female patient. The induction period can be described according to 2 types of kinetics: during the first phase (<6h), PCT increased by approximately 0.5 ng/ml per hour after a latency phase of about 2–3 hours (first measurable value recorded at time = 3h) followed by massive PCT production at the rate of approximately 50 ng/ml per hour over subsequent hours (40).

The effect of cytokines on PCT induction

The extent to which PCT can be induced *in-vivo* by individual pro-inflammatory mediators has not been fully elucidated. There is considerable evidence to confirm induction of PCT by cytokines and other factors. In addition to experimental studies on isolated cells, clinical observations show that PCT can also be induced by factors other than bacterial endotoxins, *e.g.* TNF-α and IL-2 (22,136,180).

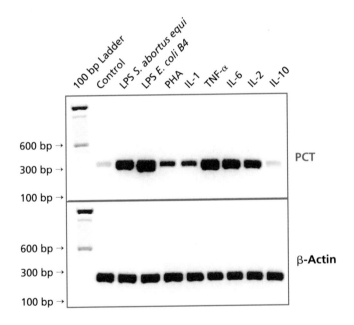

Figure 2.4.3

RT-PCR analysis of PCT and β-actin mRNA in cultures of human peripheral mononuclear cells following stimulation with various bacterial endotoxins, proinflammatory cytokines and phytohemagglutinin (PHA) (129).

Marked PCT elevation has been observed in patients receiving TNF-α immune therapy beneath a limb tourniquet after unwrapping the tourniquet. Similar observations were made with IL-6.

There is additional evidence of PCT induction occurring independently of bacterial endotoxins based on observations that PCT levels are elevated following heatstroke (16), acute burns (43, 164), in multiple trauma patients (77, 113, 167), in newborn infants (45) and after primarily sterile surgery (88, 100, 103, 104). PCT is increased within 6 hours in patients with burns without any measurable concentrations of endotoxins or TNF-α (43). There were no clinical signs of bacterial infection in these patients during the early phase of their clinical course.

Based on knowledge acquired to date, however, bacterial toxins are by far the most potent stimulator of PCT induction.

Stability and kinetics

The stability of PCT in blood samples

Unlike most cytokines, PCT is highly stable in collected blood samples. *In-vitro* plasma PCT concentrations fall by approximately 12% at room temperature and by 6% at a temperature of 4°C over the 24-hour post-collection period (111). PCT can thus be collected with routine laboratory specimens without any need for special storage conditions. The samples should be stored in a refrigerator or, if storage or transport times are prolonged or if any additional influence on the samples is to be avoided during the scope of the studies being implemented, deep frozen until required for analysis. Both the type of anticoagulation and the use of plasma or serum have no effect on PCT measurements. However, a standardized collection technique, anticoagulation process and storage procedures should be used for each hospital in order to minimize any discrepancy in the values obtained (111).

Kinetics and half-life of PCT *in-vivo*

PCT induction is very rapid. PCT levels increase in response to a stimulus within 2–6 hours (see chapter 2.4). Following an initial increase, the decline in PCT values depends on the balance between the plasma half-life and on new PCT production.

A half-life of approximately 20–24 hours is expected for PCT after a single, acute stimulus. This was determined by means of the endotoxin experiments in healthy subjects (46, 85, 137) and after accidental administration of a bacterially contaminated solution for infusion (40). Under clinical conditions, the elimination half-lives have been determined to lie within a higher range in many cases (101, 172). The elimination half-life of PCT is not significantly prolonged in patients with impaired kidney function (101, 172).

In patients with septic shock, plasma levels remain high due to on-going PCT production. A fall in plasma levels to 50% of the initial concentrations has been reported after an average of 2.4 days in patients who recovered from septic shock. Elevated levels lasted for 27 days in patients with a fatal outcome (126).

Based on our experience, a fall of more than 30% in PCT values compared with the previous day is correlated with a clinical improvement in septic patients (108). This decline should, however, be observed over several days (at least three days) (see chapter 3.3).

PCT reacts much more rapidly than C-reactive protein both in terms of the time to onset of induction and in the interval between improvement in clinical conditions and a clinically interpretable fall in values (106, 107, 109, 114).

The length of time to PCT synthesis and the type of induction show that the production of PCT is closely correlated with inflammatory activation and is related to the induction of proinflammatory cytokines. This correlation has been confirmed by clinical data (127). According to current investigations, secondary induction of PCT by proinflammatory cytokines is feasible although they are not the principal stimulus of PCT induction under clinical conditions. Recent studies in mononuclear blood cells show that TNF-α and other cytokines induce PCT mRNA. Bacterial endotoxins are the most potent stimulus for PCT induction in this system (129). The clinical relevance of *ex-vivo* measurements has not yet been confirmed as the cells tested do not release any noteworthy quantities of PCT (94, 171).

The course of PCT, CRP, TNF-α and IL-6 following experimental stimulation with endotoxin

Following intravenous administration of bacterial endotoxin, PCT levels increase after the induction of TNF-α and IL-6. Once the peak values of TNF-α and IL-6 have been reached, PCT plasma levels rise sharply after a latency period of approximately 2 hours following the initial stimulus. TNF-α and IL-6 reach peak concentrations about 1.5 hours and 2 to 3 hours respectively after the endotoxin challenge (see also Figure 2.6.1). Peak PCT values are reached within 12–48 hours in the form of a plateau. 48 to 72 hours later, the values slowly start to decline (Figures 2.4.1 and 2.4.2). In comparison, plasma concentrations of C-reactive protein (CRP) could not be detected 6 hours after administration of endotoxin, as shown in the studies conducted by Assicot (7). A similar PCT kinetic profile was reported by F.M. Brunkhorst in a female patient given an accidentally bacterially contaminated solution for infusion and after chest surgery (Figures 2.4.2, 2.6.1) (40, 175).

The clinical course of PCT and cytokines

There is a similar correlation in the time course of PCT, IL-6 and TNF-α during the acute course of clinical infections as demonstrated in the afore-mentioned experimental studies. With acute infections, PCT levels mirror IL-6 and TNF-α values after a few hours (Figure 2.6.1) (127, 175). Zeni *et al.* reported a clinical correlation between PCT and TNF-α as far back as 1994 (169) in patients presenting with severe sepsis and septic shock (r = 0.477, p = 0.0067, n = 27, Spearman correlation). If the inflammation rapidly wanes, PCT values start to decline after a decrease in IL-6, but noticeably before the decline in CRP values.

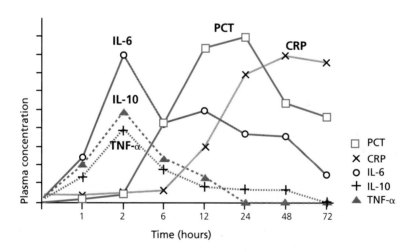

Figure 2.6.1

Time course of plasma concentrations of procalcitonin, C-reactive protein and cytokines after surgical trauma. Schematic representation (175).

In subacute and chronic inflammation, the kinetics of PCT may differ considerably from those of IL-6, TNF-α and CRP. In such cases, cytokine concentrations fluctuate far more than suggested by the clinical picture. In contrast, PCT has a much better correlation with the course of the disease than is the case with cytokines or even CRP (see case reports and chapter 3 entitled "Sepsis, shock and multiple organ dysfunction syndrome").

PCT as a surrogate marker

Oberhoffer *et al.* (127) investigated the statistical correlation between plasma PCT levels and TNF-α and IL-6 cytokines. Both CRP and PCT values were significantly correlated with TNF-α and IL-6. The probability of detecting a certain concentration of TNF-α or IL-6 was greatest with PCT levels. Values of 0.81 and 0.79 respectively were calculated for the area under the curve (AUC) on determining the probable predictive significance of a TNF-α concentration of over 40 pg/ml and IL-6 value in excess of 500 pg/ml using the "Receiver-Operating Characteristics" (ROC) technique. The corresponding values for CRP were 0.73 and 0.72 and for leukocytes and body temperature the values were considerably below 0.6.

Only slight downregulation of PCT

In contrast to the plasma concentration course followed for cytokines, downregulation is generally not observed with PCT. Current clinical experience indicates that PCT values remain considerably above the normal range even after prolonged sepsis. Lower values may, however, be observed in individual cases during courses of protracted, severe diseases without there being any marked improvement in clinical condition. Should the infection recur, plasma PCT levels normally increase.

In experimental studies in healthy subjects, repeated endotoxin injections did not produce a fall in PCT concentrations 72 hours after the first stimulus (1, 8, 9) (Figure 2.4.1). This should classified as a potential downregulation. These studies suggest that the absence of a cytokine or TNF-α response could be involved as a potential co-stimulant of PCT to the endotoxin challenge. A marked downregulation of TNF-α and other cytokines is known to occur after repeated administration of endotoxin.

Even in cases of protracted, systemic inflammation, PCT levels are generally responsive to induction stimuli. PCT levels therefore, are able to provide a better evaluation of clinical course compared to TNF-α, IL-6 or CRP. Apart from downregulation in response to repeated stimuli, TNF-α and IL-6 often react non-specifically and present considerable fluctuations in daily levels suggesting temporary activation or suppression of the immune reaction. This lack of specificity and daily variation in levels make a clinically relevant assessment difficult. CRP also shows a similar high level of variability and non-specificity. Additionally, elevated CRP values are observed in most cases even after the acute inflammatory reaction has started to wane. CRP values also peak to their maximum concentration already during the less severe stages of septic disease. Therefore, little additional information is available from subsequent measurements during the course of the disease, especially in the case of an aggravation of the disease. PCT has a significantly greater correlation with the clinical course of sepsis than the other parameters discussed above.

Immunological properties

Numerous factors suggest that PCT is of functional significance in the immune response. Arguments supporting this hypothesis include the direct time correlation of PCT increase to a corresponding inflammatory event, the rapid synthesis kinetics of PCT and the specificity of induction by proinflammatory stimuli. Furthermore, PCT levels increasing in conjunction with a florid bacterial infection have also been observed. Experimental studies support the hypothesis of an immunological or immunomodulatory effect of PCT.

PCT as a lethal factor in the laboratory animal shock model

Laboratory animal experiments in the hamster have clearly shown the potential functional significance of PCT in terms of immune response. The studies were conducted by Nylen *et al.* in bacterially induced septic shock in hamsters and published in Critical Care Medicine (123). The mechanisms of action and the type of interaction via which PCT interferes with immunological functions could not be elucidated in these studies.

Nylen *et al.* triggered bacterial-induced septic shock in the hamster by intraperitoneal administration of *E. coli.* In this animal model, PCT neutralisation by means of specific anti-PCT antibodies significantly reduced mortality. Fatality was 6% compared with 62% in the control group following prophylactic administration of the antibody ($p < 0.0001$, log-rank test). A significant reduction in mortality was also observed when the PCT antiserum was administered one hour after infection induction. A fall in the mortality rate of 82% was observed in the control group compared with 54% in the treated group ($p < 0.022$, log-rank test). Although experimental administration of human PCT to healthy animals did not trigger any toxic effects, an increase in mortality from 56% to 93% was observed with concomitant induction of bacterial shock and administered human PCT (30 µg/kg) ($p = 0.02$, log-rank test) (Figure 2.7.1).

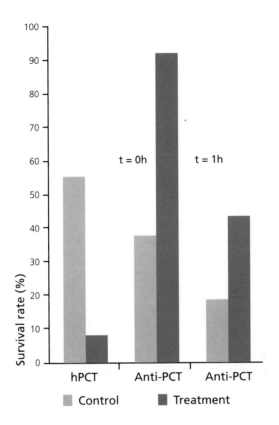

t = 0h   t = 1h

Survival rate (%)

hPCT   Anti-PCT   Anti-PCT

■ Control   ■ Treatment

Figure 2.7.1

Procalcitonin as a potential lethal factor in a hamster model of bacterial shock. Administration of human PCT increased the mortality rate in this model (hPCT group) whereas anti-PCT-effective antibodies exerted a protective effect. The latter is evident following prophylactic (anti-PCT group, left) or therapeutic application (anti-PCT group, right). The anti-PCT-antibody is not administered to the therapeutic group (right) until one hour after the endotoxin challenge via i.p. application of bacterial pellets with 5×10^8 colony-forming units of *E. coli* 018:K1:H7 (according to 123).

No detection of specific immunological effects

Regardless of these studies, our own working party investigated the effects of synthetic PCT on various immunological systems *in-vitro*. The initially assumed inhibitory effect of PCT on eicosanoid metabolism could not be confirmed with various preparations of PCT and the use of specific anti-calcitonin and anti-katacalcin anti-bodies. The effect of PCT on eicosanoids and on cyclic-AMP is less marked than that of salmon calcitonin (31).

Direct stimulation of cytokines by PCT was not observed in these studies. Inducible nitric oxide formation is supposedly reduced under the influence of PCT (177).

A slight, yet significant modulation of endotoxin-stimulated production of TNF-α and IL-6 by synthetic PCT was observed in whole human blood (31, 150). TNF-α and IL-6 secretion was inhibited by approximately 20–30% by PCT compared with the non-exposed control. Also in a hamster *in-vivo* model, PCT did not stimulate a cytokine response itself, however in septic animals, PCT injection slightly diminished IL-1β production 3 hours after PCT injection (180). These values fluctuate in a range in which an immunologically significant effect *in-vivo* is unlikely.

Further evidence of a possible modulatory effect of PCT on immunological functions is the observation of calcitonin binding sites on T- and B-lymphocytes (99). Calcitonin receptors induce G-protein mediated intracellular activation including elevation of intracellular cAMP levels and activation of phosphatidylcholine-specific phospholipase C (PC-PLC) which is an important key enzyme for the activation of inflammatory processes (55,58).

PCT has potential intracellular functions

Computer-aided analyses of amino acid and DNA sequences highlight the potential functions of PCT. These are, however, purely hypothetical and must be confirmed by functional and biochemical studies. Potential sites of phosphorylation as well as sequence homology to tubulin-binding proteins can be found on the protein sequence of PCT. According to the author, PCT may also be involved in the regulation of vasomotility or interfere with nitrogen monoxide (NO) mediated pathophysiological effects. There is, however, no experimental proof to corroborate this hypothesis which must, for the time being, remain speculative. Regardless of these studies, binding of anti-katacalcin antibodies to vascular endothelia as well as to other cells and tissues was observed following immunohistochemical staining of sections of tissue from septic patients (94). Binding was also observed in the region of the microtubular cytoskeleton of cells (171). However, given the limited specificity of these immunological test techniques, these observations must be supplemented by additional, more specific procedures.

Potential hormonal effects: calcium and phosphate metabolism

Laboratory animal experiments conducted in the hamster have shown that calcium and phosphate concentrations in the blood change during experimentally induced sepsis and these changes are correlated with an increase in calcitonin immunoreactive proteins (including PCT) (159). A fall in serum calcium values and an increase in phosphate concentrations were observed in this model. The clinical data are, however, inconsistent and cannot always confirm the results obtained in the animal model. Nylen et al. reported an increase in calcium and phosphate levels (120) in patients suffering from pneumonia. Modified serum calcium values and phosphate levels were also reported in severe forms of malaria although no direct correlation with PCT was established (47, 48).

When discussing functional aspects of PCT, it is worth noting that functional groups on the calcitonin protein sequence may be fixed functionally to katacalcin or N-PCT via coupling. On the other hand, it can be assumed that PCT also forms a ring structure with disulfide bridges (cystein 1-7 in the calcitonin sequence). At calcitonin, the ring structure is obviously not essential for receptor activity (168) but a loss of N-terminal amino acids reduces receptor activation whereas affinity to the receptor is largely maintained. This should be considered when comparing the tertiary structure of PCT with that of calcitonin.

Phylogenetically, the presence of a stable prohormone in several animal species suggests that PCT might be of considerable functional importance. Until now inflammatory induced PCT could not be detected in all animal species.

PCT in various body fluids

The question of PCT concentrations in various body fluids is often posed. Brunkhorst *et al.* (41) measured PCT levels in various body fluids in order to obtain information relating to the origin of PCT and to use potentially locally increased production of PCT as a marker for local infection of the corresponding compartment or organ.

No increase in PCT production in special compartments

The answer to the question of specific induction of PCT in various body compartments must be answered negatively. There is no specific PCT increase in special body fluids such as the CSF in meningitis, ascites in peritonitis or pleural fluid or broncho-alveolar lavage in pneumonia. The PCT content of these body fluids is low even when PCT plasma concentrations are high. Ascites fluid is one exception to the observations to date. In this instance, the concentration was approximately two-thirds that of the concentration of plasma PCT and never exceeded those of the plasma. According to studies conducted by Leon *et al.* (92), there is a correlation between PCT levels in pleural effusion and PCT serum concentrations.

PCT values measured in urine fluctuate over a wide range. Depending on the concentration of the urine, PCT values both substantially below and close to plasma levels have been observed. On average, approximately 25% of the plasma concentrations can be detected in the urine (172). Kidney function does not have a significant effect on the plasma elimination rate of PCT and plasma PCT levels (101, 172).

We have also measured PCT concentrations in ultrafiltrate during hemofiltration. PCT elimination could be measured in the ultrafiltrate using a polysulfone membrane (Baxter Renaflo® II PSHF 1200, a frequently used filtration membrane) (sieving coefficient = 0.24). According to studies conducted to date, this filtration is also devoid of a significant effect on the extent and elimination rate of plasma levels. This also applies to hemodiafiltration (174).

It should be noted that the standard measuring technique with the LUMItest® PCT test kit cannot be used alone when measuring PCT from body fluids other than blood plasma or serum. Depending on the nature of the sample to be measured, either "zero serum" must be added or a "recovery method" involving the addition of a defined quantity of PCT to an additional sample be used and a control measurement taken.

3   Sepsis, shock and multiple organ dysfunction syndrome (MODS)

3.1   Complications of infection: sepsis and septic shock

One of the more frequent and most important indications for PCT determination is the monitoring of patients at risk of infection. PCT accurately detects the systemic complications of bacterial infections. The onset of severe sepsis cannot be documented as effectively using traditional parameters as it can with PCT. Increased PCT values are an alarm for the timely detection and treatment of sequelae of disease. Regional perfusion and microcirculation disorders, coagulation disorders or metabolic changes often lead to multiple organ dysfunction syndrome (MODS).

There is a good correlation between PCT and inflammation activity and the severity of sepsis. The parameter is thus effective for monitoring the course of disease and therapy in sepsis and MODS. If the systemic inflammation exceeds that of a normal immune response due to an infection, PCT induction is rapid and predictable. Plasma levels rapidly fall as the inflammatory activity regresses.

PCT detects the highly significant systemic complications of an infection

Unlike other parameters with a high differentiation probability, PCT levels correlate with complications of infection such as the onset of organic dysfunction or metabolic phenomena and can thus be used to detect "severe sepsis" or "septic shock" (77, 131, 169) (Figure 3.1.4). The terms "severe sepsis" and "septic shock" refer to the definition of sepsis according to the criteria of the 1992 Consensus Conference [ACCP/SCCM criteria (5), Figure 3.1.1]. Only neopterin was found to possess properties similar to those of PCT in a few studies. This parameter is, however, also induced in non-bacterial inflammatory diseases. PCT is also increased in protracted shock of non-bacterial etiology (cardiogenic shock, shock during MODS) (49, 181, 105). In these situations, PCT is assumed to be induced due to bacterial translocation and proinflammatory cytokines.

Definition of sepsis according to ACCP/SCCM criteria

According to the definition of the 1992 ACCP/SCCM criteria (5), "sepsis" is a complication of bacterial infection characterized by the systemic inflammatory response syndrome ("SIRS"). Initially there is no evidence of organ dysfunction or arterial hypotension ("shock"). Changes characterized by organ dysfunction or shock symptoms appear only in cases of "severe sepsis" or "septic shock". In European terms, the concept of "sepsis" denotes the generally severe forms of sepsis which, based on ACCP/SCCM criteria, are referred to as "severe sepsis" or "septic shock". In this document, the term "sepsis" will be based on the definition given in the ACCP/SCCM criteria. The latter are defined in Figure 3.1.1.

Correlation with the severity of sepsis

Initial data relating to a correlation between PCT and severity of sepsis were published by Zeni in 1994 (169). One hundred and forty-five patients admitted to the emergency department with suspected infection were evaluated in this study and classified according to the bone criteria of septic shock (5, 28) (4 groups). Increasing PCT values were recorded in patients presenting with more severe symptoms of sepsis (Figure 3.1.2).

Definitions of systemic inflammation and sepsis according to the criteria of the Consensus Conference of the American College of Chest Physicians/Society of Critical Care Medicine (ACCP/SCCM)

Systemic Inflammatory Response Syndrome "SIRS"

At least 2 of the following criteria must be satisfied:
- Fever or hypothermia
  - Core temperature >38°C or <36°C
- Tachycardia
  - ventricular rate >90 bpm
- Tachypnea or hyperventilation
  - >20 breaths/min or PaCO2 <4.3 kPa (<32 mmHg)
- Leucocytosis or leukopenia or left-shift in differential blood count
  - 12 G/l or <4 G/l or immature/total neutrophil granulocyte count >0.1

"SIRS" with non-infectious etiology
"Sepsis": symptoms of SIRS and infectious etiology

"Severe sepsis"
Symptoms of sepsis
and
- *Organ dysfunction*
and
- *Hypotension*
  - arterial systolic blood pressure <90 mmHg
  - fall in BP values of more than 40 mmHg
or
- *Hypoperfusion with systemic phenomena*
  - lactic-acidosis
  - oliguria
  - CNS symptoms
  - other organ manifestations

"Severe sepsis": "sepsis" + organ dysfunction

"Septic shock"
"Sepsis" or "severe sepsis"
and
- *Hypotension*
  - despite fluid intake
and
- *Hypoperfusion*
  - as in "severe sepsis"

"Septic shock": sepsis/severe sepsis + hypotension (catecholamine required)

Figure 3.1.1

Systemic inflammation and sepsis criteria according to the definition of the ACCP/SCCM Consensus Conference (1992) (5, 67). Slight PCT induction, if any, is observed solely with SIRS symptoms (2, 3 or 4 criteria according to ACCP/SCCM with no infection detected). "Severe sepsis" and "septic shock" are, however, characterized by impaired organ perfusion, arterial hypotension and metabolic changes. In this instance, PCT induction is particularly marked.

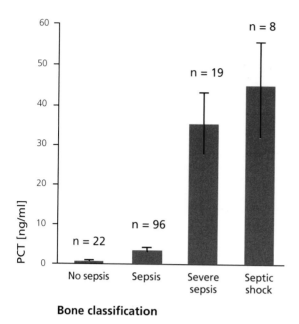

Figure 3.1.2

Correlation between PCT and the severity of sepsis. The sepsis classification based on the bone classification criteria (5, 28) (4 groups) shows markedly higher PCT values in patients presenting with more severe symptoms of sepsis (according to 169). n = No. of patients.

According to studies conducted by Gramm *et al.* (personal communication) in 63 patients with systemic inflammation and infection, only the APACHE III score, PCT and neopterin could differentiate significantly between the diagnosis of SIRS and "severe sepsis". Parameters such as CRP, IL-6, IL-8, IL-10, leukocyte count and elastase were far less accurate (Figure 3.1.3). Investigations conducted by other authors have corroborated these results (77, 125, 131).

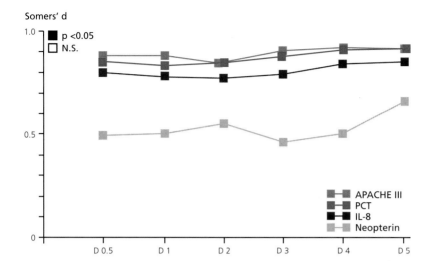

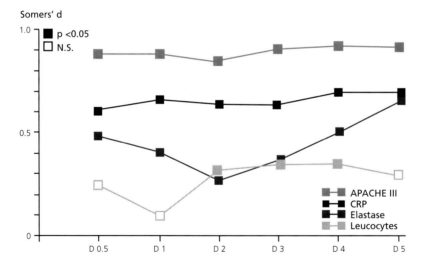

Figure 3.1.3

Statistical values to distinguish between "SIRS" and "severe sepsis". Correlation coefficient values (0 to 1) of Kendall's rank correlation are displayed, D = day (H.-J. Gramm *et al.*, with the kind permission of the author).

Only PCT and neopterin differentiate between "sepsis" and "severe sepsis"

The complications of sepsis with metabolic and functional organ dysfunction and thus the transition to "severe sepsis" or "septic shock" is characterized by a highly significant rise in PCT levels. The traditional parameters of inflammation and infection cannot differentiate between these stages of sepsis to any significant degree (77, 125, 131).

The distinction between "SIRS" and "sepsis", however is not always clear-cut with PCT. According to the studies conducted by Oberhoffer *et al.*, C-reactive protein (CRP) provides additional information for the differential diagnosis of "SIRS" versus "sepsis". This confirms the observation that, compared with PCT, CRP reacts to infections of minor severity and is therefore "more sensitive". The disadvantages of increased sensitivity however include non-specific induction and the fact that CRP values have already exceeded their range in sepsis and septic shock and can therefore provide little additional information (105). CRP also reacts more slowly than PCT, regardless of whether values rise or fall. All the other parameters investigated such as TNF-α, IL-6 or PMN-elastase were far less capable of distinguishing between the severity of systemic inflammation based on the definition of the ACCP/SCCM criteria (77, 125, 131).

The particularly high specificity of PCT for the diagnosis of severe sepsis or septic shock versus a disease associated only with the symptoms of "SIRS" or "sepsis" according to the ACCP/SCCM definitions is compared with that of other parameters in Figures 3.1.4 and 3.1.5. Corresponding data were collected in a study conducted by Lestin and Scherkus (77) (Figure 3.1.4) and Oberhoffer *et al.* (125) (Figure 3.1.5) in ICU patients. In both studies, PCT differentiated between the progression of a "SIRS"- or "sepsis"-related disease versus "severe sepsis" or "septic shock" to a significantly high degree. No other parameter effectively distinguished between these disease stages with comparable accuracy. Only neopterin possessed similar properties although this did not reach the level of significance of PCT. Differentiation based on parameters such as leukocytes, elastase, CRP, AT III, D-dimers and lactate is feasible only in isolated cases. Similar results were obtained in the studies conducted by Gramm *et al.* (Figure 3.1.3).

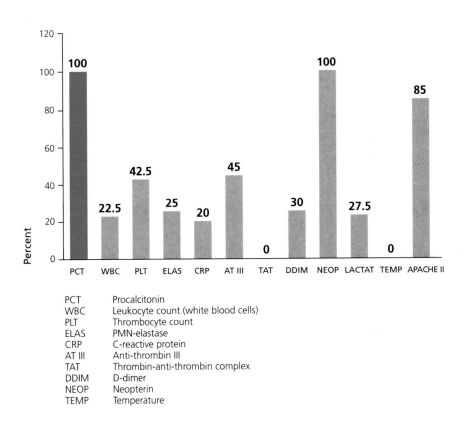

PCT	Procalcitonin
WBC	Leukocyte count (white blood cells)
PLT	Thrombocyte count
ELAS	PMN-elastase
CRP	C-reactive protein
AT III	Anti-thrombin III
TAT	Thrombin-anti-thrombin complex
DDIM	D-dimer
NEOP	Neopterin
TEMP	Temperature

Figure 3.1.4

The probability of distinguishing between SIRS and sepsis including severe forms of sepsis is between 90 and 100% for PCT and neopterin. Only a sporadic differentiation of these diseases is feasible with traditional parameters (77, with the kind permission of the author).

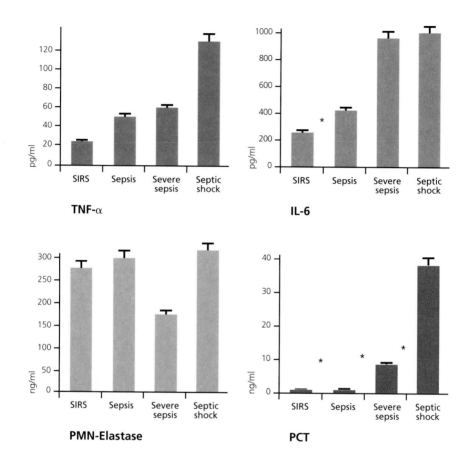

Figure 3.1.5

Comparison of the plasma levels of TNF-α, IL-6, elastase and PCT with increasing severity of systemic inflammation and sepsis according to ACCP/SCCM criteria (data recorded in 100 patients cared for in an ICU for over 48 hours). * p <0.05 (M. Ober-hoffer, reproduced with the kind permission of the author).

Is there a limit value for the diagnosis of severe sepsis?

According to studies carried out by Gramm *et al.* (personal communication), the cut-off point for the diagnosis of severe sepsis and septic shock is 5.5 ng/ml PCT with a sensitivity of 81% and a specificity of 94% for the diagnosis of generalized inflammation. PCT values ranging from 5–10 ng/ml have also been proposed by other authors as an important limit value for the diagnosis of severe systemic inflammation secondary to infection (61, 75, 77, 87, 158). According to Hammer (158) and Lestin (77), PCT plasma concentrations in excess of 10 ng/ml are almost exclusively indicative of generalized infection. When plasma concentrations reach these levels, the diagnosis should be re-assessed and specific therapy instituted. Since values are bound to differ given the varying etiology of the diseases in various patient groups and in different specialist fields, the results of individual studies are listed in Table 3.1.1.

Table 3.1.1

PCT in diseases of varying severity characterized by symptoms of systemic inflammation or infection. The range of PCT values and their sensitivity and specificity in the corresponding diagnoses are listed.

Disease severity	PCT [ng/ml] Statistical distribution	No. of patients
1 SIRS	0.6 ± 2.2	215
2 SIRS + infection	6.6 ± 22.5	53
3 Septic shock	34.7 ± 68.4	20
	Mean ± SD	
1 Pneumonia (out-patients)	0.2 (0.1 – 6.7)	149
2 Peritonitis	3 (1.1 – 35.3)	14
3 Sepsis	31.8 (0.5 – 5420)	85
	Median (range)	
1 Severe bacterial pneumonia	2.4 ± 3.7	
2 Cardiogenic shock	1.4 ± 1.9	7
3 Septic shock	96 ± 181	7
	Mean ± SD	15
1 No sepsis	0 – 1.5 (range)	30
2 Septic shock	112 (37 – 441)	39
	Median/quartile	
1 Local/regional infection	0.3 – 1.5 11	
2 Viral infection	0 – 1.4*18	
3 Severe infection	6 – 53 19	
	(range)	
1 Edematous pancreatitis		18
2 Sterile necroses		14
3 Infected necroses – fine needle biopsy		
1 Autoimmune diseases	<0.5	42
2 1 + infectious complication	1.9 ± 1.19	16
1 Viral meningitis	0.32 (0 – 1.7)	41
2 Acute bacterial meningitis	54.5 (4.8 – 110)	18
	Mean (range)	
Newborn infants:		
1 Not infected	0 (0 – 29)	497
2 Assumed infection	1 (0 – 27)	
3 Infection in newborn infants	11 (0 – 191)	
	Median (range)	
1 KTX with rejection reaction	KTX = kidney transplantation	13
2 KTX with infection		17

Diagnostic accuracy: sensitivity/specificity (%)	Criterion	Author	Reference
60% / 79% – 91% / 39%	PCT >0.5 (1 vs 2 + 3) PCT >0.1 (1 vs 2 + 3)	Al-Nawas	(2)
		Gramm	(68)
100% / 72% – 100% / 35%	PCT >1.5 (3 vs 1+ 2) PCT >0.1 (3 vs 1+ 2)	de Werra	(49)
100% positive, 82% negative predictive value	PCT >5	Hatherill	(75)
		Assicot	(7)
94% / 91% 87% / 84%	PCT >1.8 (3 vs 1+2) Comparison: PCT/ Fine needle aspiration	Rau	[148]
100% / 84%	Infectious complication	Eberhard	(50,51)
94% / 100% p <0.0001	PCT >5.0 for bacterial meningits	Gendrel	(61)
73% / 99%	PCT >6	Kuhn	(87)
87% / 70%	PCT >0.5	Eberhard	(52)

Correlation with disease severity

Since most, if not all, organ systems are affected in the case of severe sepsis and septic shock, very high PCT values are also evident using the corresponding score systems that describe the disease risk profile (APACHE II/III score) or the severity of organ dysfunction (*e.g.* SOFA score) (105) (Figures 3.1.6 and 3.1.7). There is, however, an indirect relationship in the correlation between PCT values indicating multiple organ dysfunction and disease severity. PCT is not a parameter for the assessment and grading of multiple organ dysfunction, but rather a parameter for the evaluation of inflammatory activity.

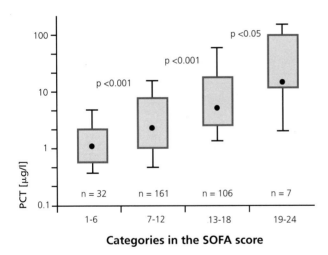

Figure 3.1.6

Distribution of PCT concentrations with varying SOFA scores in 40 patients (316 observation days) with systemic inflammation, sepsis and multiple organ dysfunction syndrome [SOFA score = Sepsis-related Organ Failure Assessment Score (162)] (105, 107).

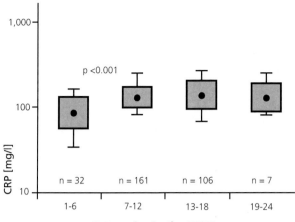

Figure 3.1.7

Distribution of CRP concentrations with varying SOFA scores in 40 patients (316 observation days) with systemic inflammation, sepsis and multiple organ dysfunction syndrome [SOFA score = Sepsis-related Organ Failure Assessment Score (162)] (105, 107).

3.2 Cardiogenic shock, circulatory dysfunction and resuscitation

PCT induction without a bacterial focus

PCT can be induced with prolonged shock of non-septic origin, *e.g.* cardiogenic shock, without any isolated bacterial focus being apparent. The values in this instance are generally lower than those expected for bacterial infections. The PCT values measured with documented microbial pathogens are on average higher than those when no pathogens are present (Table 3.2.1) (2).

Group	PCT [ng/ml], statistical distribution		
No sepsis	0.12	±	0.04
Sepsis	2.36	±	0.49
Severe sepsis	37.1	±	16.5
Septic shock	44.8	±	22
SIRS	1.3	±	0.2
Sepsis	2.0	±	0
Severe sepsis	8.7	±	2.5
Septic shock	38.6	±	5.9
SIRS	0.6	±	2.2
Sepsis (BC-)	6.6	±	22.5
Sepsis (BC+)	8.5	±	19
Septic shock	34.7	±	68.4
FUO (onset/peak)	0.75	±	1.0	(1.1 ± 1.0)
Sepsis	0.5	±	0.45	(0.8 ± 0.6)
Severe sepsis	5.8	±	8.1	(7.3 ± 8.0)
Septic shock	19.6	±	24	(37 ± 33)
Cardiogenic shock	10.1	±	15.3	(25 ± 35)
SOFA score <7	1.1		(0.6–2.4)
SOFA score 7–12	2.6		(1.3–7.7)
SOFA score 13–18	6.1		(3.0–19.9)
SOFA score >18	15.2		(12.7 – 93.1)

Table 3.2.1

PCT in patients with systemic inflammation, sepsis and MODS. Higher scores are observed with increasing disease severity. Values are expressed as the mean ± standard deviation (SD) or standard error of the mean (SEM) or median and 25%–75% percentile. BC = blood culture, FUO = fever of unknown origin.

PCT induction without any apparent bacterial focus is feasible considering that high concentrations of proinflammatory cytokines and other mediators can be detected in plasma with these diseases. Bacterial pathogens and endotoxins frequently can be found in the blood due to barrier dysfunction secondary to defective immune competence and regional perfusion disorders (bacterial translocation) (43, 53, 96, 139). According to studies conducted by Engelmann et al., elevated endotoxin values of over 10 pg/ml are correlated with significantly higher PCT values (endotoxin >10 pg/ml: PCT 96 ng/ml; endotoxin <5 pg/ml: PCT 6.9 ng/ml) (53).

No. of patients	Score	Reference
22 96 19 8	Bone classification (ACCP/SCCM criteria) (Mean ± SEM)	Zeni (169)
333 108 20 120	ACCP/SCCM Criteria (Mean ± SEM)	Oberhoffer (126)
215 53 49 20	Change in bone classification (Mean ± SD) BC, blood culture	Al-Nawas (2)
13 26 29 20 13	ACCP/SCCM criteria (Mean ± SD)	Brunkhorst (personal communication)
32 161 116 7	SOFA score (162) (Median, 25/75 percentile, in 4 groups)	Meisner Palmaers (105, 107)

Cardiogenic shock

In cardiogenic shock (left- or right heart failure), the PCT concentrations found initially are low (1.8 ± 4.9 ng/ml PCT) as compared to those of primary septic shock (89.5 ± 133 ng/ml) (mean and standard deviation, p = 0.0001) (36, 181). Similar observations were reported by de Werra et al with values of 1.4 ± 1.9 ng/ml PCT in cardiogenic shock and 96 ± 181 ng/ml in septic shock (mean value ± SD) (49).

In the case of prolonged cardiogenic shock of over 12 hours' duration, PCT values increase, reaching very high concentrations in the plasma similar to septic shock (36). This increase in values ("slope of the relationship between PCT concentration and time") at the start of the disease is less than that of septic shock over the same time interval (2.0 ± 3.5 ng/ml per 24 hours compared with 14.5 ± 6.4 ng/ml per 24 h, p = 0.04) (36, 181).

Resuscitation

Generally speaking, PCT is only slightly increased after resuscitation following cardiovascular failure, an exception is in the case of prolonged attempts at resuscitation (F.M. Brunkhorst, personal communication).

The slight rise in PCT values after resuscitation is possibly due to endotoxin release secondary to bacterial translocation from the intestine. As mentioned earlier, systemic inflammation may occur later due to reperfusion following prolonged circulatory collapse, thus triggering PCT induction.

In this context, it should be noted that elevated PCT values were observed after cardiac surgery when catecholamines were required to maintain adequate circulation (100, 176).

3.3   The prognostic value of PCT

One of the most important indications for determination of PCT is monitoring the course of systemically active infections and their prognostic evaluation. PCT reflects the extent of systemic inflammation secondary to infection. In cases of severe infection, the course of inflammatory factors together with the potential onset of progressive organ failure generally determines patient prognosis. PCT values quickly fall once the acute inflammation has waned whereas plasma levels fail to return to normal in the case of persistent systemic inflammation secondary to infection. PCT can therefore be used to assess the prognosis in patients with sepsis and multiple organ dysfunction syndrome and to follow up the surgical removal of a focus of infection or monitor the conservative treatment of an infection.

- Increasing or persistently high PCT values indicate ongoing inflammatory disease activity and suggest a poor prognosis.

- Declining values indicate a diminishing inflammatory reaction, successful removal of the infectious focus and thus a favorable prognosis.

Increasing or decreasing PCT values can therefore be crucial in deciding whether or not further diagnostic procedures are required and for modifying or confirming therapeutic interventions. Determination of PCT has economic consequences as well. Further diagnostic procedures can be dispensed with following the surgical removal of an infectious focus if PCT values fall rapidly after surgery whereas unchanged, high values indicate that additional diagnostic procedures should be conducted and a new therapeutic approach or alternative procedure should be considered.

Prognostic evaluation of therapeutic-surgical procedures (focus removal)

A significant decrease in PCT values was observed within 3 days of the surgical removal of the focus of infection in patients who recovered from sepsis and peritonitis compared with pre-surgical values (67, 68). PCT values fell from 19.0 ng/ml (median) to 7.5 ng/ml (p <0.001, n = 14) (67). No significant decrease in PCT values was observed in patients who died (n = 16). In this case, values increased or stayed at the same level. Plasma concentrations averaged over 10 ng/ml (Figure 3.3.1).

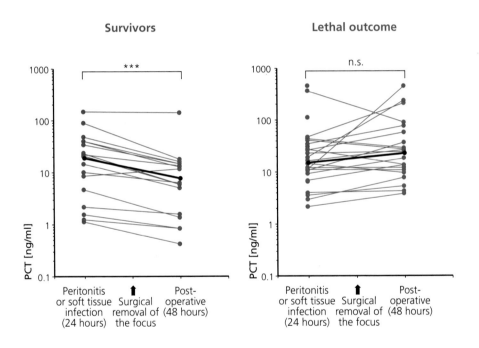

Figure 3.3.1

Plasma PCT concentrations in patients who recovered (n = 17) or died (n = 25) from peritonitis or soft tissue infection (sepsis) after having undergone surgical removal of the focus (*** p <0.001, n.s. = not significant; Wilcoxon test) (68).

Comparable results were reported in a larger patient population (n = 246) (146). In the case of peritonitis, PCT values significantly decreased within 48 hours after surgery in patients with a favorable prognosis. In cases with a fatal outcome, however, PCT values either increased or stayed the same. Peritonitis was due to perforation of a cavity organ in 78 patients, to pancreatitis in 44 patients and to another cause in 38 cases. PCT concentrations differed significantly on the first, fourth and last day of the observation period (p <0.05). No significant differences were recorded as regards CRP (146).

Prognostic evaluation in peritonitis

PCT predicted the outcome of the disease with 84% sensitivity and 91% specificity in a prospective study involving 162 patients presenting with peritonitis (144). This was based on assessment of the course of PCT plasma concentrations between Days 0 and 3. The inclusion criteria on Day 0 were as follows: clinical signs of peritonitis, assisted ventilation and a Hannover-Intensive score of 8–12 points. Decreasing values between Days 0 and 3 were observed in patients whose condition improved whereas unchanged or increasing values indicated a fatal outcome. No significant difference was observed between groups in TNF-α and IL-6 levels or the APACHE II score.

Assessment of the clinical course and prognosis of sepsis

The course and follow up of PCT values is important for assessing both the clinical course of the disease and its prognosis in sepsis or systemic inflammation (67, 68, 108, 112, 141, 144, 146). Massive induction of PCT indicates severe systemic inflammation secondary to bacterial infection with an increased risk of fatality. A limit of 10 ng/ml PCT is considered by many authors to be a more reliable indicator of severe infection with the symptoms of systemic inflammation (77, 158). Regardless of any surgical procedure, decreasing PCT values suggest a good prognosis.

Oberhoffer *et al.* observed persistently high PCT values in patients presenting with a fatal disease course whereas, in favorable prognoses, the values fell by 50% compared with baseline values within a matter of days (126, 146). Compared with other inflammatory parameters, PCT was the most important factor for determining the outcome in ICU patients in a study that also evaluated interleukin-6, TNF-α and CRP. The cut-off value with 80% specificity for a fatal outcome was 1.6 ng/ml (131).

The prognostic significance of elevated PCT values must, however, be considered from different perspectives. The absolute peak of initial PCT plasma levels is not always associated with a poor prognosis. High PCT values have been reported in some studies at the onset of disease with a lethal outcome (126, 141) whereas this observation could not be corroborated in another patient population (105). Specific treatment can therefore be successful, even with very high PCT values, depending on the etiology of the dis-

Group/disease	Type of assessment	No. of patients
Peritonitis	Course over Days 0–3	162
Severe abdominal infections	Course over Days 1–3	42
Sepsis, severe sepsis, septic shock	Time interval up to 50% of the baseline	56 22
Sepsis, MODS	Course over Days 1–3 based on 4 criteria or: Day 1: PCT >10 ng/ml	44
Peritonitis	Course over Days 0–3	246

Table 3.3.1

Course criteria for the prognosis of systemic inflammation and sepsis. Sensitivity and specificity data pertaining to various criteria.

ease. Prognostic evaluation based on changes in plasma PCT levels is therefore preferable to the assessment of individual values and the initial peak PCT value.

Prognostic evaluation based on changes in PCT values

An attempt was made to identify factors based on clinical experience that affect the course of PCT levels in order to increase the prognostic value of the changing levels. It was determined that, in addition to the actual level, the extent and duration of the change, *i.e.* the kinetics, are also important (108). Corresponding studies carried out in order to assess PCT values are summarized in Table 3.3.1. Common to all studies was the finding that a decline in PCT levels over several days correlated with successful removal of the infectious focus and a good prognosis.

Statistics	Criterion	Author	Reference
58% sensitivity 72% specificity On course assessment: 84% sensitivity 91% specificity	PCT >10 - lethal course. Increasing or unchanged values during course assessment: lethal course	Reith	(144)
Level of significance: p <0.001 (Wilcoxon test)	Decreasing PCT values indicate patient survival	Gramm	(67, 68)
2.4 days (survival) 27 days (lethal course)	A 50% decrease compared with baseline values	Oberhoffer	(126)
85% sensitivity 85% specificity or 33% sensitivity 87% specificity	4 criteria for end point assessment survival/death or: initial PCT value >10 ng/ml	Meisner, Palmaers	(105)
84% sensitivity 91% specificity	Increasing or unchanged PCT values: lethal course	Reith	(146)

Diagnostic and therapeutic consequences

Determination of PCT has diagnostic and therapeutic consequences. This applies not only to cases in which a bacterial focus is suspected or the effectiveness of antibiotic treatment assessed. If an infectious focus has not been detected, a rise or fall in PCT values can be interpreted as an increase or decrease in inflammatory activity. This can influence a decision to modify the diagnostic plan or to continue or adjust a specific therapy.

Determination of PCT also has economic consequences in terms of financial and material resources. Even the administration of antibiotics can be governed by PCT. However, in this case it should be noted that antibiotics may also be required in patients with normal PCT levels since PCT levels are typically not increased with localized infections.

The guideline should be to direct diagnostic and therapeutic activities on the basis of various diagnostic tools and the overall clinical impression of the patient. A single parameter cannot replace this procedure but can, however, constitute an important "stepping stone" in this approach. PCT therefore "sounds the alarm" in situations which are difficult to diagnose.

PCT following removal of the focus

Once a bacterial focus has been removed, normal PCT values indicate that a generalized infection is no longer present and that systemic inflammation is under control. A residual local bacterial focus cannot, however, be ruled out. Antibiotic therapy or further surgical procedures may therefore be required until no further clinical signs of infection are apparent (142).

Clinical course assessment via PCT levels

The course of PCT values during sepsis reflects the increasing or decreasing systemic immune reaction of the body. PCT values often run parallel with the patient's clinical condition and give early confirmation of a successful therapy or improvement in the patient's disease (see also the case reports in Figures 3.4.1 and 3.4.3). In many cases, a rapid decline in elevated PCT values towards normal levels is associated with an improvement in the clinical condition (chapter 3.3) (68, 144). On the other hand, if PCT values change only slightly over time or remain at a pathological level (e.g. >2 ng/ml), then this finding is generally synonymous with the ongoing critical condition of the patient (Figures 3.4.2 and 3.4.4). In fatal outcomes, PCT values often rise prior to the final stage. Studies carried out to investigate the relationship between the clinical course and prognosis and PCT levels are presented in Table 3.3.1.

Special features during an acute clinical course

During an acute course, it should be noted that at high PCT values, i.e. during an episode of marked PCT induction, levels must naturally fall. This initial drop in very high PCT levels should not be overestimated. The course of PCT values should thus be monitored over several days.

Special features of a prolonged clinical course

In some patients, a prolonged clinical course is characterized by low, albeit above-normal and occasionally declining PCT values with little or no change in the clinical condition of the patient. Typically only minor inflammation is evident in these patients. In such cases, a bacterial or inflammatory focus may also be present. Low PCT values can therefore indicate general exhaustion of the immune system ("PAID", post-aggression immunologic depression) and down regulation of the immune system. In these cases, ongoing treatment should be specific and clinically orientated.

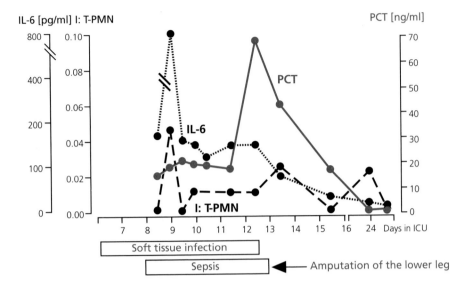

IL-6 [pg/ml] I: T-PMN

PCT [ng/ml]

Soft tissue infection

Sepsis ◀— Amputation of the lower leg

Figure 3.4.1

A 23 year-old male patient with multiple trauma and open fracture of the lower leg. The patient presented with septic symptoms on Day 8 after admission, obviously due to soft tissue infection. During the subsequent course, elevated PCT levels indicated a marked exacerbation of the inflammatory reaction. The patient's condition improved following amputation of the lower leg. (I:T-PMN = ratio of immature neutrophil granulocytes to the total granulocyte count) (H.-J. Gramm, Benjamin Franklin Clinic, FU, Berlin).

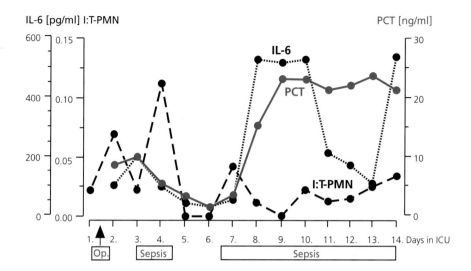

Figure 3.4.2

65 year-old male patient with peritonitis after perforated diverticulitis of the sigma. The course of increased PCT values correlates with the clinical diagnosis of sepsis and indicates that local therapy was unsuccessful (I:T-PMN = ratio of immature neutrophil granulocytes to total granulocyte count) (H.-J. Gramm, Benjamin Franklin Clinic, FU Berlin).

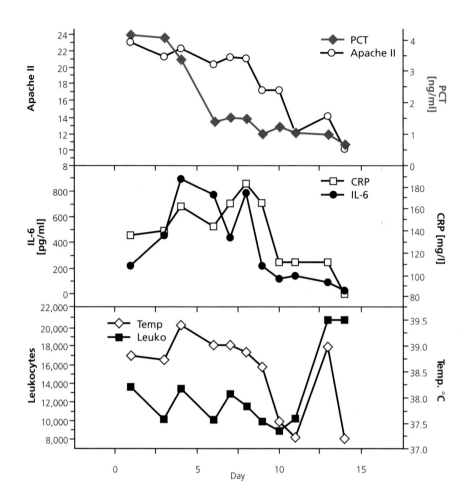

Figure 3.4.3

Successful operation performed on a perforated ileum with subsequent peritonitis. The 35 year-old female patient was discharged from the ICU on post-operative day 14 (102).

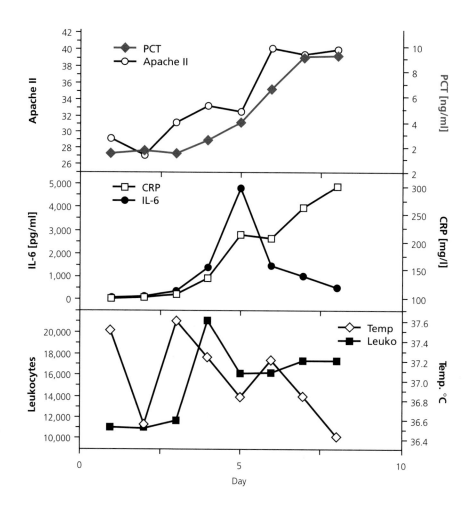

Figure 3.4.4

70 year-old female patient with resection of the chest wall and necrotic tissue due to local infiltrating, superinfected carcinoma of the breast. Complete surgical elimination of the infected tissue was not possible due to the extended, infiltrated local findings, as reflected by PCT values which did not fall after surgery. The subsequent continuing rise in PCT levels emphasised the poor prognosis. The patient died on postoperative day 8 (102).

3.5 A comparison to parameters of the inflammatory response

Numerous inflammatory induced parameters are available for the diagnosis of inflammatory diseases. In addition to the differential blood count, these include acute phase proteins such as C-reactive protein (CRP), inflammatory mediators such as cytokines including interleukin-6, interleukin-8 and TNF-α or other parameters such as neopterin, elastase and phospholipase A_2.

Each of these parameters has a specific induction profile and its own characteristics in various forms of disease. These values are compared with PCT in this monograph.

The results of individual studies can be used to highlight the differences between important inflammatory parameters and PCT, especially in sepsis and systemic inflammation. The results of studies in which PCT was compared to other parameters are listed in tables at the end of this chapter (Table 3.5.1).

Although this illustration is incomplete, it nevertheless shows that PCT offers an advantage over parameters established to date particularly in septic diseases (Figure 3.1.3). PCT provides greater specificity than cytokines or other parameters in the differential diagnosis of bacterial and non-bacterial diseases, *e.g.* in transplantation medicine, autoimmune diseases or acute infectious diseases.

The fundamental differences between PCT and cytokines

Cytokines are function proteins that fulfil a specific immunomodulatory function. Naturally, the half-life and stability of most cytokines are relatively low to trigger rapid reactions to changes in the patient's immunological status. High peak values may therefore appear and subsequently quickly disappear over a short time span. This is a disadvantage as far as clinical diagnosis is concerned as the validation of normal values is compounded and the diagnostic window reduced.

"Maintenance" or "memorizing" of the induced values is guaranteed in a clinically relevant range through the beneficial *in-vivo* half-life of PCT which is approximately 24 hours. The clinical course of plasma PCT concentrations is therefore stable and readily interpretable.

The rise in PCT kinetics is only slightly delayed compared with cytokines (Figure 2.6.1). PCT is therefore also suitable for acute diagnosis. CRP reacts much more slowly than PCT. This point should be kept in mind when interpreting inflammatory parameters.

Unlike cytokines, PCT is also very stable in whole blood, plasma or serum even at room temperature. Thus samples do not generally have to be refrigerated immediately. The high stability of PCT in the blood samples collected means that this parameter can easily be used in routine clinical diagnosis without measurements being adversely affected during storage and transportation.

Another advantage of PCT compared with cytokines is the relative specificity of PCT for bacterial- and septic-induced inflammation. With many cytokines, other events of minor impact on disease progression or prognosis may trigger a very high yet transient rise in values.

Table 3.5.1

Comparison of PCT to various inflammatory induced parameters during various diseases. The mean and standard deviation are presented for PCT, CRP and IL-6 and other parameters, unless stipulated otherwise. PCT (ng/ml), CRP (μg/ml), IL-6 (pg/ml), neopterin (nmol/l), elastase (μg/l), TNF-α (pg/ml), NO_2/NO_3 (mM).

Study/patient population	PCT	CRP
Differential diagnosis		
Pancreatitis: non-infected vs. infected necrosis: cut-off, sensitivity/specificity (%)	1.8 ng/ml 94.4% 90.6%	300 μg/ml 83.3% 81.2%
Pancreatitis: Toxic etiology Biliary etiology	0.39 ± 0.38 60.8 ± 136	96.6 ± 97.5 173 ± 126
ARDS: Non-infectious etiology Infectious etiology	0.6 ± 0.95 36.6 ± 31	180 ± 146 179 ± 122
Urinary tract infection Pyelonephritis	0.38 ± 0.19 5.37 ± 1.9	30.3 ± 7.6 120 ± 8.9
Sepsis and shock		
SIRS (ACCP/SCCM criteria) Sepsis "Severe sepsis" "Septic shock" *p <0.05 compared with the next easiest stage	1.29 ± 0.2(SE) 2.03 ± 0* 8.71 ± 2.5* 38.6 ± 5.9*	128 ± 3 160 ± 6* 193 ± 11* 160 ± 6*
		NO_2/NO_3
Bacterial pneumonia Cardiogenic shock Septic shock (Days 0 and 1)	2.4 ± 37 1.4 ± 1.9 96 ± 181	37 ± 28 26 ± 13 72 ± 60
Sepsis: 1st day (mean, SD) Survival Fatal outcome	4.9 ± 2.9 13.8 ± 8.9	223 ± 65 245 ± 72
Cardiogenic shock (after 24 h) Septic shock (after 24 h)	2.0 ± 3.5 14.5 ± 6.4 p = 0.04, (MW test)	20.8 ± 41.3 19.8 ± 34.9

IL-6	Other parameters	No.	Author	Reference
No data	IL-8: 112 pg/ml 72.2% / 75%	50	Rau	(141)
645 ± 792 723 ± 848	Neopterin: 8.7 ± 11 45.6 ± 41	22	Brunkhorst	(38)
704 ± 789 856 ± 890	Neopterin: 13.5 ± 7.32 229 ± 225	17	Brunkhorst	(37)
No data	Leukocytes: 10939 ± 834 17429 ± 994	60	Benador	(21)
269 ± 22 435 ± 52* 69 ± 168* 996 ± 57	TNF-α: 24 ± 4 51 ± 9* 59 ± 17 118 ± 18	333 108 20 120	Oberhoffer	(125, 134)
10 ± 13 78 ± 74 385 ± 251	TNF-α: 32 ± 17 11 ± 13 108 ± 132	29	de Werra	(49)
434 ± 198 443 ± 178	TNF-α: 38 ± 16 42 ± 21	236	Reith	(141)
269 ± 38 0.8 ± 2.7 p = 0.001 (MW test)	Neopterin: 9.8 ± 20.1 26.8 ± 61.2	55	Brunkhorst	(36)

Table 3.5.1 (continued)

Study/patient population	PCT	CRP
Transplantation		
Kidney transplantation: Sensitivity/specificity for the diagnosis of an infection	87% 70%	100% 43%
Autoimmune diseases:		No data
No infection	0.5 (<0.9)	
Infection	1.3	
(median, 25/75 percentile)	(1.1–2.5)	
Children and newborn infants		
Meningitis:		
Viral	0.32 ± 0.35	14.8 ± 14.1
Bacterial	54.5 ± 35.1	144 ± 69
Severe viral infection	0.28 (0–1,5)	
Localised bacterial infection	1.7 (0.1–4.97)	
Invasive bacterial infection	29.7	102
(mean, range)		

Cytokines are generally subject to marked down regulation mechanisms. PCT is relatively insensitive to these influences.

In certain situations, *e.g.* autoimmune diseases or in transplantation rejection, diagnosis of systemic infection with cytokines is not feasible as stimulation has already occurred within the framework of the underlying disease. Thus the differential diagnostic properties of PCT are not observed in this context with cytokines and other parameters, as confirmed by the results obtained by various authors (33, 35, 37, 39, 75, 141, 73, 74).

IL-6	Other parameters	No.	Author	Reference
No data	No data	57	Eberhard	(52)
	No data	324	Eberhard	(50)
No data	No data	59	Gendrel	(61)
		120	Gendrel	(62)
850				

Comparison of selected cytokines: IL-6 and IL-8

IL-6 is a highly reliable parameter for characterizing the immune response in severe diseases. IL-6 values correlate relatively well with the extent of the immune response and disease severity. Moreover, IL-6 is more stable than TNF-α. However, unlike PCT, cytokines IL-6 and TNF-α are also induced non-specifically, e.g. during transplantation rejection, after surgery, in viral infections and in autoimmune diseases. A relatively marked fluctuation in IL-6 levels is observed compared to PCT concentrations and distinct down regulation can be observed with IL-6. Out of 290 patients with sepsis, only 75% presented with detectable IL-6 levels (70). More recent studies have confirmed the proportional rise in IL-6 values in line with sepsis severity (125, 134). In the sepsis study with monoclonal anti-TNF-antibody fragment MAK 195F

(143), high IL-6 values were considered to be an indicator for a subgroup of patients with marked hyperinflammatory components and were therefore used as a treatment inclusion criterion.

Which parameter (IL-6 or PCT) is best suited for various disease conditions must be investigated depending on the indication. PCT was far superior to IL-6 in assessing the prognosis of peritonitis and IL-6 levels did not suggest any significant difference between surviving patients and a fatal course (144). In transplantation rejection, only very high IL-6 values are considered indicative of an infection. IL-6 concentrations are, however, suppressed by steroid therapy, but not those of PCT (158). In the case of burns, PCT is equal to IL-6 as a marker for evaluating the severity of tissue damage (43). PCT offers additional advantages compared to IL-6 for the differential diagnosis of bacterial diseases. According to studies conducted by Brunkhorst et al. (35, 37, 38), no significant differences were observed for IL-6 in patients with ARDS and pancreatitis of varying etiology.

PCT is also obviously superior to IL-6 in assessing the course and prognosis of sepsis. At the beginning of the disease, IL-6 and IL-8 are closely associated with the extent of generalized inflammation (42). However, the correlation decreases as the disease progresses. IL-8 plasma concentrations differ significantly in patients with disease of infectious and non-infectious etiology (98). Less sensitivity and specificity were observed for IL-8 in contrast to PCT in patients with infected necrosis in pancreatitis compared to sterile necrosis or edematous pancreatitis (141). According to the results of a study conducted by Oberhoffer et al., PCT (1.6 ng/ml), IL-6 (280 pg/ml), TNF-α (24 pg/ml) and CRP (198 mg/l) were the most important factors for determining outcome in ICU patients. In this study PCT had the greatest correlation with the outcome (131).

TNF-α

TNF-α is involved in the onset of sepsis or MODS but TNF-α plasma levels are of little relevance for diagnostic purposes. According to the data obtained in several studies, TNF-α levels can be detected in less than 50% of all patients presenting with sepsis (148). Furthermore, there is only a slight correlation with disease outcome (148) and differentiation between "SIRS" and "sepsis" cannot be confirmed by TNF-α. The sensitivity and specificity of soluble TNF-α receptors for the diagnosis of sepsis are greater than those observed with TNF-α but less than those of PCT (49). In all comparisons of TNF-α and PCT, diagnosis has proved less certain and less reliable with TNF-α.

Comparison of CRP and PCT

CRP is an acute phase protein that is synthesised in the liver. Unlike the situation with PCT, a relatively minor inflammatory reaction is sufficient to stimulate CRP. Like PCT, CRP is induced by infection, and bacterial infection in particular. CRP can also be used to monitor the course of infections. In severe infections, sepsis and MODS, however, CRP has the disadvantage of being more sensitive and more non-specific than PCT. Enhanced diagnostic sensitivity compounds specificity in terms of the diagnosis of infections. CRP plasma levels are induced by viral infections, acute rejection reactions following transplantation and non-specific stimuli, e.g. surgery. These values may remain high over a prolonged period. According to the results of studies conducted by Gramm et al. (H.-J. Gramm, personal communication) in multiple trauma patients, CRP values were significantly elevated in infection-free patients even on discharge from the ICU. Conversely, PCT values in the same patient population were, on average, only slightly above the normal range of 0.5 ng/ml throughout the patients' stay. Concentrations were no longer in the pathological range on discharge.

The increased sensitivity of CRP can be beneficial in certain situations but in the case of ICU patients, it poses a distinct disadvantage. In addition, CRP values in patients presenting with sepsis, septic shock and MODS quickly reach or exceed their maximal range (105) (Figures 3.1.6 and 3.1.7). This precludes quantitative evaluation, even in the case of relatively minor symptoms of sepsis, and the clinical course cannot be reliably predicted (106, 107, 109, 125).

CRP has a slower kinetic profile than that of PCT. The plasma half-life is approximately 24 hours, but CRP production in the liver generally continues for several days, sometimes longer, even after the inflammatory stimulus has waned, so that improvement of the inflammatory situation is not evident from low plasma values. The fact that CRP is induced more slowly than PCT (>12 h) poses less of a disadvantage. The delayed kinetic profile of CRP is understandable from its function. In fact, CRP does not tend to convey as a humoral signal protein like the cytokines but forms part of the immunological defence system instead. CRP is an opsonin that is capable of activating the complement system by conventional means (135). It is also capable of binding the C-polysaccharide of Pneumococci. CRP is formed secondarily, *i.e.* the synthesis of CRP in the liver can be stimulated by IL-6 (class 2 acute phase protein).

In contrast to PCT, CRP increased 48 hours after surgery in surviving patients displaying, on average, consistent to slightly increasing values in the prognostic evaluation of peritonitis (146). A significant fall in values was, however, observed with PCT. In another patient population, both IL-6 and CRP failed to differentiate between a fatal outcome in patients with peritonitis and a favorable improvement in the clinical condition (144).

Phospholipase A₂ (PLA₂)

PLA_2 is an enzyme that cleaves phospholipid-acylester bonds (138). PLA_2 thus releases arachidonic acid from membrane phospholipids. This is also the starting product of eicosanoid synthesis. PLA_2 is thus a key enzyme in inflammatory activation. LPS induces increased PLA_2-II plasma activity. PLA_2- is induced primarily by bacterial infections but also by viral diseases (117, 148). No studies comparing PLA_2 with PCT have been carried out to date.

Elastase

Elastase is a serine proteinase derived from the azurophil granulae of neutrophil granulocytes. Elastase can cleave various plasma proteins (81). As with neopterin, elevated elastase values have been observed in cases of sepsis and correlated with mortality rates (59, 133, 165). Like PLA_2, elastase cannot distinguish between SIRS and sepsis (165). According to the investigations of Oberhoffer et al. (125, 134), there is no significant difference in plasma elastase concentrations at various stages of sepsis and SIRS defined on the basis of ACCP/SCCM criteria.

Neopterin

Neopterin is a degradation product of guanosintriphosphate and is produced chiefly by interferon-γ-stimulated monocytes. It is therefore also an indirect marker of the activity of cytotoxic T-lymphocytes (69). Neopterin values tend to follow the same pattern as those of PCT (35, 37, 77). However, neopterin is less specific for bacterial diseases than PCT. Levels can be high, particularly in the case of viral diseases, tumours and other non-bacterial diseases (158). Neopterin is thus less suitable than PCT for the diagnosis of transplantation rejection.

The fact that neopterin plasma levels depend on kidney function restricts the use of neopterin in ICU patients presenting with sepsis and MODS. However, neopterin can distinguish between fatal courses and survival in patients with sepsis (133, 165).

Neopterin can also differentiate between SIRS or sepsis and severe sepsis or septic shock with greater statistical accuracy.

At the present time, neopterin is used primarily as a more sensitive indicator for the activation of the monocytic and lymphocytic system, *e.g.* as a screening parameter for blood donors. Viral infections and HIV infections in particular react early with neopterin induction even prior to serological test conversion.

HLA-DR

HLA-DR is a monocyte-surface antigen that supposedly displays "immune paralysis" or the restricted immunological response capacity of monocytes. An inverse relationship of HLA-DR with PCT levels has been reported (83). This correlation is not, however, apparent in all patients and there are septic patients presenting with high PCT values and low HLA-DR values as well as patients who, despite a high proportion of HLA-DR-positive cells exhibit relatively low PCT levels even over a prolonged period. The extent to which "hyperinflammatory phases" or "immune paralysis" can be correlated with PCT and HLA-DR has not yet been sufficiently elucidated. However, a correlation or inverse relationship between the two parameters cannot, in any way, be accepted as a rule of thumb. Whether a hyper- or hypoinflammatory septic phase can be detected or defined by both parameters has not yet been established, similar to the definition of both conditions.

Other parameters

Leukocyte counts, differential blood counts, the erythrocyte sedimentation rate and increased body temperatures are also indicators of inflammatory activity. These parameters can be highly sensitive for any typical inflammation, however, they are rather nonspecific (77, 131), as demonstrated in Figures 3.1.6 and 3.1.7 in the ratio of immature to mature granulocytes. Their diagnostic value is thus often limited in intensive and surgical medicine (54, 131, 134).

In this context, PCT values once again reflect an improvement or deterioration in the patient's condition in severe forms of sepsis and septic shock. This is usually impossible with other inflammation parameters such as leukocytes, body temperature, CRP or cytokines. In cases of severe sepsis, the diagnostic value of these parameters is usually limited due to their overall stimulation whereas PCT is still capable of modulation.

4 Specific indications for PCT determination

4.1 Prognosis and clinical course of peritonitis

Patients with peritonitis generally present with very high PCT values. This may be due to the fact that the peritoneum has a very active immune response and that peritonitis is virtually always accompanied by signs of systemic inflammation. Since the peritoneum has a large well capillarised surface, peritonitis can rapidly spread, triggering a life-threatening infection in close proximity to the systemic circulation. In focus-limited peritonitis or locally confined peritoneal irritations such as the onset of appendicitis or cholecystitis, PCT concentrations increase only slightly if at all.

Peritonitis and sepsis

The peak PCT values occurring over the course of the disease in patients with peritonitis or pneumonia without concomitant signs of systemic inflammation are displayed in Figure 4.1.1 and compared with the respective disease with symptoms of systemic inflammation, *i.e.* sepsis according to ACCP/SCCM criteria (68). In the case of sepsis, maximal PCT concentrations are generally higher than those observed in patients with locally confined infections.

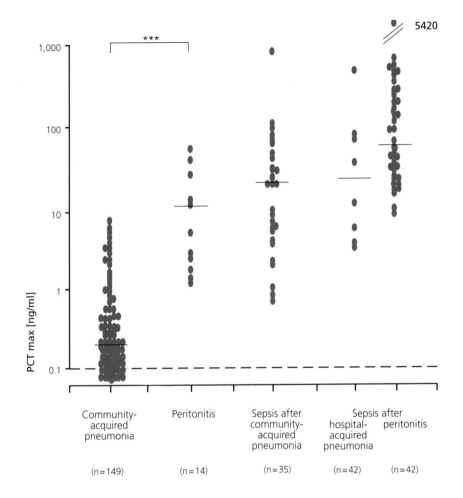

Figure 4.1.1

Serum procalcitonin concentrations in pneumonia and peritonitis with and without septic symptoms (maximal values). The bars indicate the mean of each group. The mean values recorded in the pneumonia and peritonitis groups (columns 1 and 2) are significantly different (Mann-Whitney Test, p <0.001) (68).

Monitoring the clinical course of peritonitis

In peritonitis, PCT has value as a prognostic marker. In a study conducted by Reith et al. (144) and involving 162 patients with peritonitis, it was possible to distinguish between a lethal course of the disease and those patients with a favorable prognosis with 84% sensitivity and 91% specificity. The group of patients who survived was characterized by declining PCT values from Day 0 to Day 3 whereas in non-survivors with peritonitis, PCT values increased or remained unchanged over the same period.

The results of this study were confirmed by another prospective study (146) and by data collated by Gramm et al. (68) (see also chapter 3.3).

4.2 PCT in the post-operative period

PCT values may increase during the first few days after surgery, depending on the nature and extent of the surgical procedure. A sterile surgically treated wound does not provide sufficient stimulus for PCT induction whereas major operations or intestinal procedures may trigger PCT. PCT concentrations generally lie within or slightly above the normal range after minor or primarily aseptic surgical interventions. After extended surgery, however, and abdominal surgery in particular, slight to moderately elevated PCT values are frequently observed during the post operative period but rarely exceed 2 ng/ml (88, 100, 103) (Figures 4.2.1, 4.2.2 and 4.3.4).

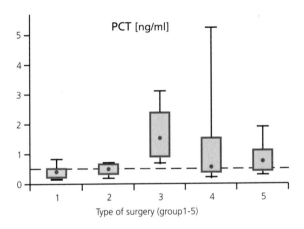

Figure 4.2.1

Maximal post-operative PCT values after various types of surgery without any complications. The observation period lasted for up to 5 days after surgery. The mean, 25/75% percentile (box) and 10/90% percentile of the respective maximal PCT values are displayed. Group 1 (n = 37), more minor procedures (inguinal hernia, total hip replacement, thyroidectomy, peripheral vascular surgery); Group 2 (n = 11), more minor abdominal interventions (cholecystectomy); Group 3 (n = 22) more complex abdominal surgery (resection of the colon, sigma, rectum, gastrectomy); Group 4 (n = 16) extended abdominal or retroperitoneal procedures (esophageal resection, Whipple's operation, major vessels); Group 5 (n = 32) cardiac and thoracic surgery (103).

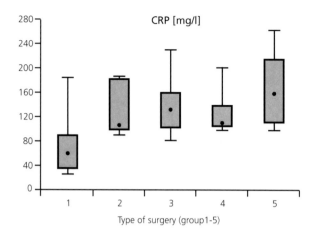

CRP [mg/l]

Type of surgery (group1-5)

Figure 4.2.2

Maximum CRP values (mg/l) observed depending on the type of operation performed as in Figure 4.2.1.

Trauma-induced increase in PCT levels

During a prospective study carried out between 1996 and 1997, PCT values were recorded before and daily after surgery up to the 5th post-operative day in 117 patients with an uncomplicated, post-surgical course and no evidence of infection or systemic inflammation (103). The results show that post-operative PCT production depended primarily on the nature and extent of surgery, but rarely exceeded 2 ng/ml. Values of up to and over 6 ng/ml were, however, observed in individual cases following more complex procedures. In many cases, these patients were characterized by the onset of delayed complications (145, 147). Maximal PCT values generally occurred between 1 and 2 days after surgery, but peak values could also be recorded at a later date (Figure 4.2.3). In virtually all cases, maximal CRP values were not reached until the 2nd post-operative day (Figure 4.2.2). Since a post-operative increase in CRP values is observed almost without exception in comparison to PCT values, the diagnostic utility of this parameter is limited during the post-operative period. PCT induced in polytraumatic patients has also a prognostic value (see chapter 4.4).

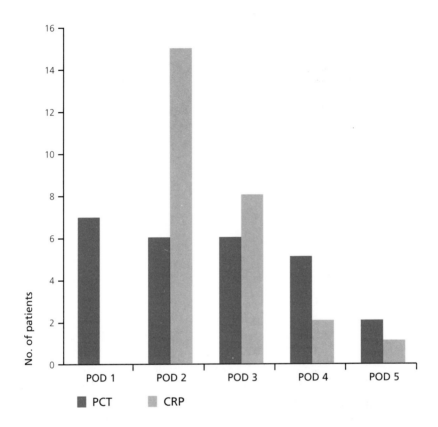

Figure 4.2.3

The day on which maximum PCT or CRP values were obtained are presented in terms of frequency of distribution in this histogram. 26 patients were examined up to the 5th day after cardiac surgery (POD 1-5) (100).

Minor surgery and primary aseptic operations

Whereas only 32% of patients presented with PCT values higher than 0.5 ng/ml and just 3% with values in excess of 2.0 ng/ml following minor surgery such as cholecystectomy, closure of an inguinal hernia or primary aseptic procedures such as artificial hip replacement, thyroidectomy and peripheral vascular surgery, 59% of patients presented with PCT values above the normal range of 0.5 ng/ml and 11% above 2 ng/ml following cardiac surgery (Figure 4.2.4) (100, 103, 110). The time course of post-operative plasma PCT concentrations following cardiac surgery is shown in Figure 4.2.4 (103).

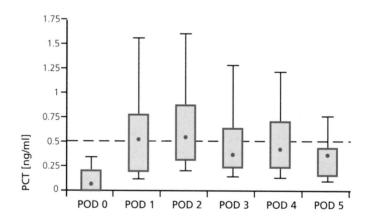

Figure 4.2.4

The time course of PCT values (ng/ml) following cardiac surgery with extracorporeal circulation (bypass surgery, valve replacement, n = 26). The mean value, 25/75% percentile (box) and 10/90% percentile are depicted; POD = post-operative day (100).

Major surgical procedures and abdominal operations

Elevated plasma PCT levels are observed in the majority of patients following abdominal surgery. Values over 0.5 ng/ml were recorded in 65% of patients undergoing abdominal operations (small intestine, colon, sigma or rectum resection, gastrectomy, n = 20). Twenty-five per cent (25%) of patients presented with values of over 2 ng/ml and one patient had concentrations over 5 ng/ml (5.13 ng/ml). High values were also measured with similar frequency after extended abdominal or retroperitoneal procedures (aortic aneurysm, Whipple's operation, esophageal resection). The maximum value recorded in these cases was 5.7 ng/ml. PCT values averaging 2.1 ng/ml and ranging from 0.9 to 8.2 ng/ml PCT were also recorded by Marnitz et al. in patients with esophageal resection (n = 7) (97).

PCT in cardiac and thoracic surgery

PCT values are also slightly elevated following cardiac and thoracic surgery. According to our own studies (100, 103), the mean value obtained after cardiac surgery with extracorporeal circulation was 0.74 ng/ml. 90% of patients presented with values below 1.77 ng/ml PCT (n = 25). Corresponding values of 0.58 ng/ml and 1.64 ng/ml were observed in comparable thoracic operations without extracorporeal circulation (n = 12) and did not, therefore, differ from procedures involving extracorporeal circulation. The patients did not develop any complications and there was no evidence of inflammation (SIRS criteria). Values of this order were also reported by Hensel et al. (76). In this study, PCT values of 0.9 ± 1.0 ng/ml were observed in patients devoid of symptoms of SIRS (n = 23). The PCT concentrations did not differ significantly in cases with symptoms of systemic inflammation (n = 8). Significantly higher PCT values were recorded only in patients with acute lung failure (8.0 ± 2.7 ng/ml, n = 9). Kilger et al. (84) compared post-operative PCT values following conventional coronary artery bypass surgery with heart-lung machines and after minimal invasive bypass surgery without extracorporeal circulation. Virtually no PCT was induced due to the minor surgical trauma following the minimally invasive technique (mean 0.7 ng/ml PCT, n = 27).

Potential causes of post-operative PCT induction

The cause of elevated post-operative PCT values has not yet been determined. Both transient intraoperative bacterial contamination or endotoxin release caused by intestinal anastomoses, bacterial translocation after extracorporeal circulation or during extended abdominal or retroperitoneal interventions may be factors. Other pro-inflammatory mediators such as IL-6 and TNF-α, both of which are known to occur following major surgical trauma, may also trigger PCT induction.

The implications for diagnosis

Recognition of raised PCT values following surgery is important for the interpretation of post-operative PCT levels. It should be noted that the nature and extent of the individual operation will have a marked influence on the level and frequency of post-operative PCT induction. Early determinations should therefore be undertaken in risk groups or following major surgery to identify post-operative risks and to distinguish between infection- or sepsis-induced PCT induction and increased post-operative values secondary to surgical trauma.

According to studies conducted by Reith et al. (145), a PCT value which exceeds 1.5 ng/ml on the first or second post-operative day is an indicator for subsequent potential complications. Post-operative PCT values of this magnitude therefore suggest close monitoring of the patients in question or continuation of antibiotic therapy. If PCT values are used as a diagnostic parameter after surgery, routine determination from the 1st post-operative day is recommended. Only in this way can plasma PCT levels be properly documented during the post-operative course since differentiation between elevated post-operative values and a sepsis-induced increase in PCT concentrations is considerably more difficult when interpreting individual values.

Type of surgery	n		25%	median	75%	90%	Max.
1. More minor surgical procedures, primarily aseptic surgery with:	37	PCT CRP	0.18 36	0.38 61	0.55 93	0.73 181	2.5 265
– hip joint replacement	14	PCT CRP	0.37 59	0.48 91	0.56 172	1.38 183	1.59 184
– peripheral vascular surgery	15	PCT CRP	0.20 30	0.29 34	0.63 80	0.77 165	2.49 265
– thyroidectomy and hernia operation	8	PCT CRP	0.18 55	0.26 67	0.42 78		0.53 99
2. Cholecystectomy	11	PCT CRP	0.29 198	0.49 106	0.60 182	0.62 197	0.62 200
3. Abdominal surgery (colon, sigma, rectum resection, gastrectomy)	20	PCT CRP	0.80 99	1.50 131	2.31 160	3.00 230	5.13 250
4. More major surgical procedures involving the mediastinum or retro-peritoneum with:	12	PCT CRP	0.31 102	0.54 109	1.49 142	4.99 204	5.76 206
– aortic aneurysm Y prosthesis	5	PCT CRP	0.51 104	1.65 106	3.32 128		5.76 144
– Whipple's operation	1	PCT	–	–	–		0.26
– esophageal resection	6	PCT CRP	0.22 104	0.45 133	0.65 201		0.91 206
5. Cardiac and thoracic surgery	37	PCT CRP	0.38 115	0.61 161	1.24 221	1.77 261	4.96 395
with: – cardiac surgery (with extracorporeal circulation)	25	PCT CRP	0.38 124	0.74 195	1.09 241	1.77 291	2.99 395
– thoracic surgery (lung resection)	12	PCT CRP	0.31 101	0.58 133	1.61 159	1.64 228	4.96 250

Table 4.2.1

Maximal procalcitonin [ng/ml] and CRP [mg/l] plasma concentrations during a 5-day post-operative observation period in patients with a post-operative course devoid of complications. The mean and 25/75/90% percentile are listed together with the highest respective value observed (max.) (103).

Marker	ALF (%)
PCT >5 ng/ml	
Sensitivity	100
Specificity	100
IL-6 >400 pg/ml	
Sensitivity	33
Specificity	100
Neopterin >10 nmol/l	
Sensitivity	33
Specificity	75
Leukocytes >12,000/µl	
Sensitivity	100
Specificity	50
Elastase >150 µg/l	
Sensitivity	67
Specificity	30
CRP >5 mg/l	
Sensitivity	44
Specificity	13
sL-selectin >1,250 ng/ml	
Sensitivity	22
Specificity	100

Table 4.2.2

Sensitivity and specificity of post-operatively increased values of inflammatory parameters in patients with systemic inflammation (SIRS) following cardiac surgery with extracorporeal circulation in relation to diagnosis of acute lung failure (ALF) (76). In this study, 17 out of 40 patients developed SIRS after surgery, 9 of whom presented with acute lung failure [definition according to Murray *et al.* (116)]. PCT = procalcitonin, IL-6 = interleukin 6, CRP = C-reactive protein, elastase = leukocyte-elastase, sL-selectin = soluble L-selectin.

Transplantation surgery

The normal immune response of the body is pharmacologically suppressed following organ transplantation. This results from the use of corticosteroids, cyclosporin and other immunosuppressants to prevent acute transplant rejection. Bacterial, viral or fungal infections therefore represent life-threatening complications in 25% of transplantations (110). Successful organ transplantation is jeopardized by acute rejection of the transplanted organ in a further 30% of cases.

Acute organ rejections must be discriminated from infections at an early stage since these conditions require different and contradictory forms of therapy. Infection-induced symptoms can, however, be eclipsed by an acute rejection such that early, reliable diagnosis of the infection is often difficult in patients presenting with concomitant rejection.

PCT in the diagnosis of infection in patients following transplantation

PCT provides another diagnostic tool for use after transplantation. Elevated PCT levels indicate a systemic infection just a few hours after the onset of infection. PCT values of over 10 ng/ml are often observed in the case of sepsis and severe bacterial infections. Conversely, a significantly PCT release does not occur in viral infections or by an acute rejection reaction.

According to studies carried out by Staehler *et al.*, the onset of infection was detected by PCT values of >1 ng/ml with 77% sensitivity and 100% specificity in heart transplant patients (158). PCT concentrations in excess of 10 ng/ml were always associated with severe systemic bacterial infection in this patient population.

When assessing PCT values during the first few days after transplantation surgery, it should be noted that a non-specific increase in values may occur post-surgery depending on the type of operation performed (see chapter 4.2), *e.g.* after liver transplantation. The investigator therefore should establish reference ranges for every type of transplantation and be aware of PCT kinetics following surgery (74). Monitoring the post-operative course, even if PCT values are elevated initially, does not limit the utility of PCT as a diagnostic tool.

No PCT induction in transplant rejection

PCT is not induced during an acute rejection reaction. Significant PCT induction is, however, triggered after transplantation in patients presenting with infections and sepsis (52, 72-74, 88, 89, 155, 158). This applies to kidney transplantation as well as to heart and liver transplantation. Acute rejection following liver transplantation will not significantly affect the post-operative course of PCT values (88) (Figure 4.3.5a). No significant difference in relation to the control population was observed in kidney transplant patients presenting with rejection (52). PCT induction was not observed following heart transplantation in patients with viral infections and rejection reactions (73, 158). Increased PCT values were, however, observed in individual cases following partial necrosis of the transplanted organ (52) (own observations).

The early post-operative period

Slightly elevated PCT values are generally to be anticipated in some patients within the first few days of surgery (chapter 4.2) (100, 103). Early post-operative increase is more marked following liver (88) as opposed to kidney transplantation. An increase of approximately 50% compared with pre-surgical PCT concentrations was reported on the 1st to 3rd post-operative day following kidney transplantation (52). Concentrations ranging from approximately 0.8 to 5 ng/ml PCT were recorded in 50 percent of the patients (median of about 3 ng/ml). Peak values were likewise mainly observed on the 1st and 2nd day after liver transplantation. According to the studies conducted by Kuse *et al.* (88, 183), values of over 7 ng/ml (mean 5.2 ng/ml, S.E.M. ± 1.2 ng/ml) were observed. No specific data on PCT concentrations in patients experiencing a complication-free course following heart transplantation are currently available. It can, however, be assumed that the post-operative values after this type of operation do not differ fundamentally from PCT values observed after cardiac surgery (100, 103).

PCT can also be stimulated after transplantation

It has been confirmed that PCT induction following transplantation is not adversely affected by immunosupression. High dose steroid therapy supposedly does not inhibit PCT and TNF-α stimulation although IL-6 production is probably affected (52, 72, 89, 155, 158). PCT can be induced in patients with septic shock even after myeloablative therapy, *e.g.* autologous or allogenic stem cell transplantation (170).

Disruptive influences: OKT3 may trigger PCT release

A one to ten-fold increase in PCT concentrations was measured in numerous patients after OKT3 administration (52). The possibility of PCT release following administration of this antibody should be considered so that increasing values are not misinterpreted as infection. This observation supports the hypothesis that PCT is possibly formed in leukocytes (130). The systemic inflammatory reaction induced by OKT3 (1) may, however, be responsible for PCT production. PCT is not induced in every case after administration of anti-lymphocyte antibodies. Similar observations were made using anti-lymphocyte-globulin (128).

Other inflammatory induced parameters

Also other inflammatory parameters are affected by infection or an acute rejection reaction (Figures 4.3.1 and 4.3.2).

IL-6 and TNF-α levels rise during acute organ transplant rejection and following surgical trauma (Figure 4.3.2).

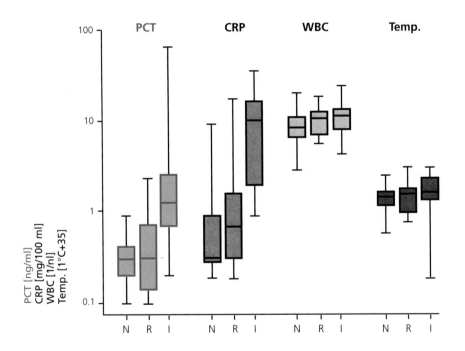

Figure 4.3.1

Kidney transplantation: Comparison of PCT, CRP and leukocyte levels and body temperature. N = regular post-operative course (n = 77); R = acute rejection reaction (at the time of biopsy) (n = 16); I = systemic infection (23 specimens). The median, 25/75% (box) and 5/95% percentile are given (Whisker); WBC = white blood cells (leukocyte count) (52).

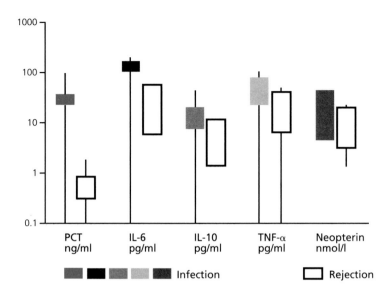

Figure 4.3.2

Mean concentrations of PCT, IL-6, IL-10, TNF-α and neopterin in 48 patients following heart transplantation and diagnosis of an infection or acute rejection reaction of
the transplanted organ (158).

IL-6 synthesis is suppressed by steroid therapy. Substantial fluctuations in concentrations over relatively short periods constitute a
further disadvantage of IL-6 measurement. Moreover, an infection can be detected with 77% sensitivity and 100% specificity
from IL-6 levels over 25 pg/ml. According to the investigations of
Staehler and Hammer (73, 158), values over 84 pg/ml rule out a
sole acute rejection reaction with 98% certainty. The data were
obtained after heart transplantation in a patient population com-
prising 96 patients.

TNF-α displays a similar pattern of behaviour to that of IL-6 but cannot discriminate sufficiently well between an acute rejection reaction, *e.g.* following heart transplantation, and an infection (158).

Neopterin increases slightly in acute rejection and markedly during infection but it can also increase noticeably in the event of surgical trauma and other non-specific incidents. Like IL-10, neopterin is therefore less suitable for the diagnosis of organ transplant rejection (155, 158).

The pre-operative phase is also important

PCT determination is also indicated in the pre-operative phase in preparation for transplantation. Transplantation must not be initiated in the event of a florid infection due to the marked initial immunosuppression. Since the pre-operative examination phase has to be very short for the transplant recipient, PCT can provide invaluable information regarding the presence or absence of bacterial infections in the time available.

An overview of key publications

Studies of PCT conducted to date and focusing on the individual types of transplantation are presented overleaf. Analysis of these studies shows that PCT has diagnostic utility which facilitates the important differentiation between a bacterial infection that can be managed with antibiotic therapy and an acute organ transplant rejection or viral infection.

Kidney transplantation

PCT values following kidney transplantation are significantly elevated in cases of invasive bacterial infections compared to patients free from infection or presenting with acute rejection without accompanying infection. According to studies conducted by Eberhard *et al.* (52) in 57 kidney transplant patients, the PCT values in 13 patients presenting with acute rejection did not differ significantly from the values recorded in patients devoid of complications ($p = 0.47$). On the other hand, PCT values were significantly increased in 17 patients with invasive bacterial infections ($p < 0.01$) (see Figure 4.3.1 and Tables 4.3.1 and 4.3.2).

Table 4.3.1

Kidney transplantation: sensitivity and specificity of PCT in distinguishing between acute organ transplant rejection and bacterial infections (52).

	PCT >0.5 ng/ml	CRP >6 mg/ml	Leukocytes >1,000/µl	Temperature >37.5°C
Specificity	70%	43%	33%	50%
Sensitivity	87%	100%	70%	17%

Table 4.3.2

Kidney transplantation: The level of significance (p) is given on the basis of the Mann-Whitney test in comparison with patients with an uncomplicated post-operative course (n = 77), acute rejection of the transplanted organ (n = 16) and a systemic infection (n = 23). The serum samples of 57 kidney-transplanted patients were used in the study (52).

Level of significance p (MWU test)	Uncomplicated course/rejection	Uncomplicated course/systemic infection	Rejection reaction/systemic infection
PCT	p = 0.47	p <0.01	p <0.01
CRP	p = 0.04	p <0.01	p <0.01
WBC	p = 0.23	p = 0.02	p = 0.65
Temperature	p = 0.10	p = 0.02	p = 0.84

The specificity for the diagnosis of an infection in this group of kidney transplant patients was 70% for PCT and 43% for CRP. As a more sensitive albeit substantially more non-specific parameter, CRP presented with 100% sensitivity compared with 87% in the case of PCT.

Langefeld *et al.* (89) reported on 20 patients who underwent kidney transplantation and 25 patients receiving liver transplants. In the case of transplant rejection (7 patients with liver transplants and 5 patients with kidney transplants), PCT values were always lower than 0.3 ng/ml. PCT concentrations ranged from 1 to 3 ng/ml in patients presenting with an infection (n = 8, pneumonia) while levels of up to 33 ng/ml were observed in cases of systemic infection (n = 5).

Liver transplantation

A post-operative rise in plasma PCT concentrations is generally always observed following liver transplantation. Kuse *et al.* (88) analysed post-operative PCT values in 40 patients following liver transplantation. Sixteen (16) patients presented with an uncomplicated post-operative course. Maximal PCT values after surgery averaged 5.2 ± 1.23 ng/ml in these patients (S.E.M., range: 1.2–15.5 ng/ml) (Figure 4.3.3). The highest values were observed on the 1st and 2nd post-operative day and declined to normal within a week. Acute transplantation rejection did not adversely affect the kinetics of plasma PCT concentrations, *i.e.* no increase in PCT values was observed (Figure 4.3.4a). In the case of infections, PCT generally responded with a marked increase in values up to 41 ng/ml (Figure 4.3.4b). Infection can thus be distinguished from rejection reactions according to the course of PCT values in many cases, even after liver transplantation (Figure 4.3.5). Differentiation achieving similar diagnostic accuracy based on traditional parameters (TNF-α, α_2-macroglobulin, etc.) was either impossible or feasible only by combining several parameters (88, 183). Increased PCT values were also observed in *Candidiasis* infection. A case report on PCT values in disseminated *Candida* infection following liver transplantation was published by Gerard *et al.* (64).

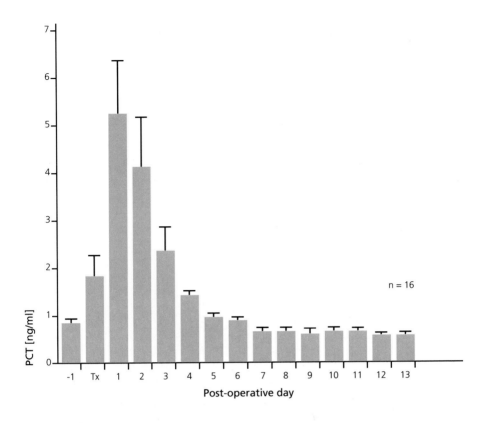

Figure 4.3.3

Course of PCT concentrations following liver transplantation with an uncomplicated post-operative course (n = 16; mean value, standard deviation from the mean) (according to Kuse *et al.*, reproduced with the kind permission of the author).

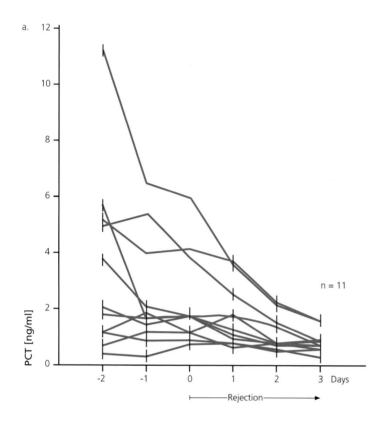

Figures 4.3.4 a-c

Time course of PCT plasma concentrations following liver transplantation.

Figure 4.3.4a: The post-operative course of PCT in 11 patients presenting with acute rejection (0 = day of diagnosis). The post-operative fall in PCT values is not affected by the rejection reaction.

Figure 4.3.4b: The increase in PCT levels is marked in 6 patients with severe systemic infections (0 = day of diagnosis).

Figure 4.3.4c: PCT increase is less pronounced in 5 patients presenting with pneumonia (according to 88).

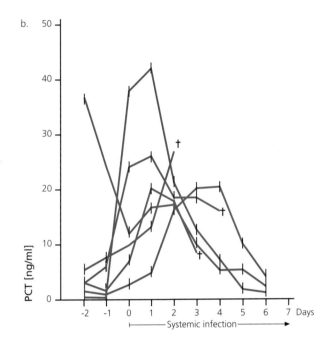

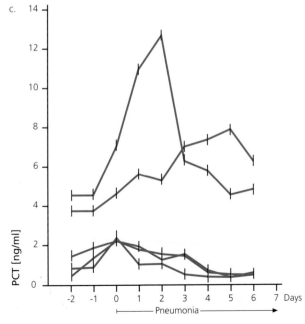

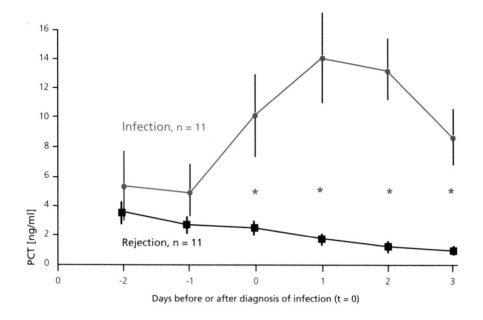

Figure 4.3.5

PCT values following liver transplantation before and after diagnosis of infection and rejection reaction (according to 88, reproduced with the kind permission of the author).

Heart transplantation

Determination of PCT can also provide important information after heart transplantation. PCT is not induced by acute organ transplant rejection while severe bacterial infections are detected by PCT (Figure 4.3.6). In the latter case, values exceeding 10 ng/ml indicate severe systemic infection (73, 74).

Staehler and Hammer from Munich published data pertaining to a group of 48 heart transplant patients, 19 liver transplant patients and 11 lung transplant patients (72, 155, 156). PCT values in patients with diagnosed bacterial infection (221 specimens) averaged 25.8 ± 4.6 ng/ml (SEM). PCT concentrations were not

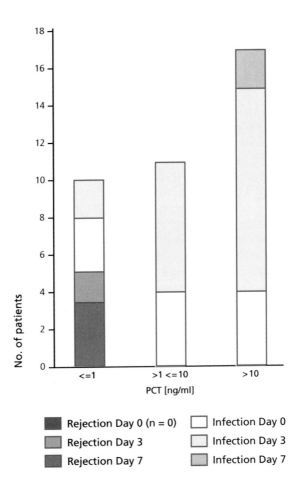

Figure 4.3.6

Correlation between PCT concentrations and the onset of infections or rejection. The data were collected in 48 heart transplant patients (158).

increased in patients with acute transplant rejection without infection (0.5 ± 0.1 ng/ml) (n = 86) compared to patients devoid of complications (PCT 0.3 ± 0.02 ng/ml) (n = 565 specimens). The authors calculated a sensitivity of 77% and specificity of 100%

(p <0.001) for the diagnosis of infection with PCT values over 1 ng/ml. Values exceeding 10 ng/ml were always indicative of severe infection. Acute rejection without concomitant infection can be ruled out with 98% certainty at this level (p <0.001).

In their studies, Staehler et al. identified the type of microbial pathogen causing the individual infections (158). The highest PCT values were recorded with generalized fungal infections. Since little information regarding the type of pathogen and level of PCT in infections has been provided so far, these data are listed in Table 4.3.3 but are not classed as representative values. The severity of the systemic inflammation and the infection were not taken into account. It is therefore feasible to assume that patients with fungal infections were suffering from a particularly severe disease as is often the case with generalized fungal infections, and PCT levels were therefore very high (73).

Table 4.3.3

PCT values in infections involving various types of pathogen. Serum PCT concentrations in 96 heart transplant patients with infections were attributed to the species of pathogen (158).

Type of pathogen	No. of measurements	PCT (ng/ml, concentration range measured)
Fungal infections (Candida spec., Aspergillus spec., Trichosporum cut.)	n = 58	0.1–334
Gram-negative rods	n = 15	0.2–260
Gram-positive cocci	n = 42	0.1 – 115
Chlamydiae and mycoplasma	n = 17	0.1 – 40
Gram-positive rods	n = 6	7.0 – 19
Pneumocystis carinii	n = 2	0.3 – 13
Viral infections	n = 6	0 – 0.1

4.4　PCT in multiple trauma patients

Increased PCT values, similar to those observed after surgery, are observed in multiple trauma patients. Values of up to 5 ng/ml are reached within the first 24 hours. Peak values generally appear within the first 12 to 24 hours. High values are frequently correlated with severe injury, injury type and prognosis (113). This correlation applies to PCT values determined within 12–24 hours after the accident.

Correlation with the severity of the injury, organ failure and outcome

According to our own studies and the results obtained by Gerlach *et al.* (personal communication), increased PCT values observed within the first 12 to 24 hours are accompanied by a higher risk of mortality. These findings support those of Mimoz *et al.* who found higher PCT levels with a more severe injury and a more frequent onset of shock and multiple organ dysfunction (113). Compared with moderate abdominal trauma, severe abdominal trauma and the delayed onset of severe pulmonary dysfunction had a significant effect on PCT values. Injuries to the extremities, chest and head as well as delayed kidney and liver dysfunction did not affect the PCT concentrations. According to Mimoz *et al.*, PCT was correlated with peak CK and LDH values and with the volume requirement during the early phase (n = 21). Once again, CRP values rise more slowly than PCT (113).

In these trauma patients, a PCT value of over 2 ng/ml 12 hours post-trauma was a strong indicator of a fatal outcome. The converse also applied—the chances of survival were high with values below 2 ng/ml. A similar conclusion could not be made with certainty based on IL-6 levels. The severity of the injury was also associated with significantly higher PCT values but not, however, with significantly elevated IL-6 values.

In terms of prognosis, multiple organ dysfunction syndrome or pulmonary dysfunction is more likely to occur in in patients with initially high PCT values.

PCT can therefore be an effective marker for evaluating the risk profile of multiple trauma patients (Table 4.4.1).

Table 4.4.1

PCT in multiple trauma patients.

- increased PCT values following multiple trauma are also possible without infection and sepsis (levels of over 5 ng/ml)
- peak values are generally reached within 24 hours
- abdominal trauma and the severity of the injury significantly affect PCT (ISS, APACHE II score)
- elevated PCT values (>1–2 ng/ml) constitute a risk factor for subsequent pulmonary dysfunction, MODS, shock and fatal risk
- there is no correlation between PCT and chest trauma, trauma to the extremities, subsequent onset of kidney or liver dysfunction.

4.5 PCT as a predictor of complications?

There is much evidence to suggest that increased, early induction of PCT following varying incidents is suggestive of subsequent potential complications. This applies to the post-operative period (chapter 4.2) (76, 100, 103, 145), multiple trauma patients (chapter 4.4) (113) as well as other diseases (chapter 4.15) (16, 43).

Are increased PCT concentrations during the post-operative period indicative of risk?

According to a study conducted by Reith et al. (145) in 35 patients undergoing colorectal surgery, post-operative PCT values during a complication-free, post-operative period averaged 1.2 ng/ml on the first day after surgery and less than 1 ng/ml PCT in 35 patients undergoing surgery to the infrarenal aorta. Early, significantly elevated post-operative PCT concentrations were observed in patients who experienced subsequent complications, e.g. pneumonia. In these patients, PCT values averaged 6.9 ng/ml in colorectal procedures and similarly 6–7 ng/ml in aorta related operations (Figure 4.5.1). Elevated, post-operative PCT values were observed as early as the first post-operative day in this study whereas the complications (e.g. pneumonia, anastomosis insufficiency, ischemia) were diagnosed clinically at a later stage [3rd to the 5th (10) day].

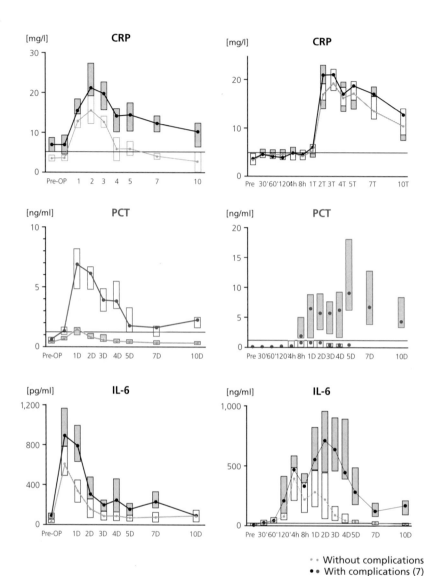

Figure 4.5.1

CRP, PCT and IL-6 concentrations in patients following colorectal surgery (left) and after infrarenal aortic surgery (right). The following levels are displayed: respective plasma concentrations in patients experiencing an uncomplicated post-operative course (white, n = 35) and post-operative complications (grey, n = 7) during the post-operative period (pre-operative to the 10th day after surgery); D, Day; (.) median; box, 25/75% percentile (145).

Increased post-operative PCT concentrations in patients with pulmonary dysfunction following cardiac surgery

PCT values of less than 2 ng/ml are generally observed after cardiac surgery in patients with a complication-free post-operative course (76, 100, 104). On the other hand, PCT values ranging from 5.1 ng/ml to 14.3 ng/ml were measured in patients presenting with pulmonary dysfunction (76). The sensitivity and specificity of other parameters determined in this study for the diagnosis of acute lung failure was markedly reduced in relation to PCT (Table 4.2.2). Additional studies should, however, be conducted in view of the low number of cases included.

We observed increased PCT values during the post-operative period in our own studies in patients predisposed to cardiac surgery risk. Thirty-seven percent (37%) of the 48 patients with a PCT value of less than 2 ng/ml developed symptoms of SIRS and 10% required catecholamines to maintain perfusion pressure whereas 61% of the 28 patients with PCT values exceeding 2 ng/ml presented with symptoms of SIRS and 68% required catecholamines. The number of patients administered antibiotics was 3-times greater in the second group compared with patients having a low PCT value (103, 104).

PCT as a risk indicator in multiple trauma

Increased PCT values occurring within the first 24 hours in multiple trauma patients (see chapter 4.4) also indicate a greater subsequent risk. Elevated PCT levels in these patients suggest the possible onset of multiple organ dysfunction syndrome and shock and indicate the frequency of pulmonary dysfunction similar to that observed by Hensel *et al.* (76) in patients having undergone cardiac surgery (see chapter 4.4).

4.6   Differential diagnosis of pancreatitis

Due to high enzymatic activity and the release of vasoactive and toxic mediators, pancreatitis can quickly develop into a life-threatening condition with multiple organ dysfunction syndrome if local complications such as pancreatic necrosis arise. The differential diagnosis of the etiology and complications associated with this disease is therefore extremely important. Rapid establishment of biliary patency is essential in the case of biliary obstruction causing acute pancreatitis. In severe cases of pancreatitis, differential diagnosis of sterile and infected necrosis will have a profound effect on the subsequent therapeutic procedure. In both cases, PCT can be an important diagnostic indicator.

According to studies published by Rau *et al.* (141), determination of PCT levels provides diagnostic confirmation similar to that of a fine needle aspiration for establishing the prognosis of infected necrosis of the pancreas. Both sensitivity and specificity are greater with PCT than IL-8. The likely prognosis of patients with infected necrosis can therefore be concluded on the basis of PCT levels. It should, however, be noted that pancreatitis is a disease associated with marked fluctuations in the degree of severity of systemic inflammation and PCT can also be induced in response to systemic inflammation.

The differential diagnosis of sterile and infected necrosis

During the clinical course of pancreatitis, the question of infected necrosis of the pancreas is relevant to disease progression and potential therapeutic measures. Fine-needle biopsy is an accurate method for the detection of infected necrosis. CT-scans without biopsy can point only indirectly to an abscess or necrosis. Since the therapeutic approach can differ in both cases (conservative therapy, abscess drainage or surgical removal of necrotic tissue), differential diagnosis will have therapeutic consequences.

The significance of PCT and interleukin-8 in the diagnosis of infected necrosis in acute pancreatitis was investigated by Rau *et al.* at the University of Ulm, Germany (141). The authors determined PCT and IL-8 in three groups of patients presenting with pancreatitis: 18 patients with edematous pancreatitis, 14 with sterile necrosis and 18 with infected necrosis. The course of PCT values compared with C-reactive protein is illustrated in Figures 4.6.1a and 4.6.1b. The markedly increased PCT values in infected necrosis (IN) compared with sterile necrosis (SN) or interstitial edematous pancreatitis (AIP) are easily recognizable as is the comparatively reduced diagnostic confirmation provided by C-reactive protein (Figure 4.6.1b) (140). With an optimized cut-off value of 1.8 ng/ml for PCT and 112 pg/ml for IL-8, which had to be reached on at least 2 days, sensitivity for the prediction of infected necrosis was 94% and 72% for PCT and IL-8 respectively with a specificity of 91% for PCT and 75% for IL-8. There was no correlation between disease etiology and the extent of the necrosis in this patient population. An uneven distribution of patients in terms of disease severity and systemic inflammation could not be ruled out in this study. Seventy-eight percent (78%) of the patients with infected necrosis presented with multiple organ dysfunction syndrome and septic complications compared with only 36% of patients with sterile necrosis and multiple organ dysfunction syndrome but no septic complications. Neither multiple organ dysfunction syndrome nor sepsis was observed in patients diagnosed with edematous pancreatitis.

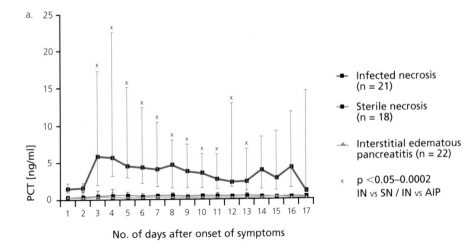

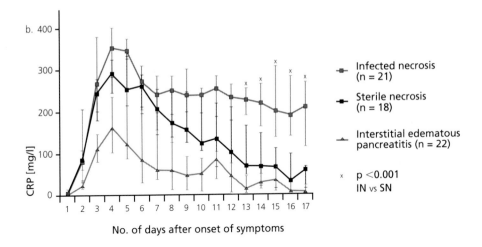

Figure 4.6.1a-b

Course of plasma PCT (4.6.1a) and CRP (4.6.1b) levels in patients with acute pancreatitis and infected necrosis, sterile necrosis and interstitial edematous pancreatitis. Significantly higher PCT concentrations were detected in patients with infected necrosis from the 3rd day after the onset of symptoms, whereas no significant difference between infected and sterile necrosis was apparent with CRP before the 13th day after the onset of disease [(140), reproduced with the kind permission of the author].

Data relating to the course of PCT and IL-8 values in patients with pancreatitis are interesting. PCT and IL-8 values observed in surviving patients following successful surgical removal of necrotic tissue fell significantly within the first three post-operative days compared with pre-surgical values whereas generally high concentrations persisted in patients with a fatal outcome. CRP failed to differentiate between the two groups (Table 4.6.1). Bertsch *et al.* (25) also reported low PCT levels on the day on which patients with edematous pancreatitis were admitted to hospital (PCT 0.69 ng/ml, mean value, n = 7) and higher values in patients with necrotic pancreatitis (sterile or superinfected, PCT 6.9 ng/ml, mean, n = 8). No further conclusions regarding infectious and sterile necrosis could be reached in this study due to the low number of cases included.

Table 4.6.1

Cut-off values for optimal sensitivity and specificity for PCT, IL-8 and CRP for the diagnosis of infected necrosis (n = 18), septic multiple organ dysfunction syndrome (n = 14) and fatal outcome of the disease (n = 11) in patients presenting with acute pancreatitis (141).

	Cut off	Sensitivity	Specificity
Predictive value: infected necrosis			
PCT [mg/ml]	≥1.8	94%	90%
IL-8 [pg/ml]	≥112	72%	75%
CRP [mg/l]	≥300	83%	78%
Predictive value: septic multiple organ dysfunction syndrome			
PCT [mg/ml]	≥3.0	86%	92%
IL-8 [pg/ml]	≥140	79%	81%
CRP [mg/l]	≥325	71%	78%
Predictive value: fatal outcome			
PCT [mg/ml]	≥5.7	100%	92%
IL-8 [pg/ml]	≥140	91%	79%
CRP [mg/l]	≥325	64%	72%

Acute pancreatitis: biliary versus toxic etiology

In acute pancreatitis, early diagnosis of biliary etiology with obstruction of the bile duct is of major significance. This is generally caused by bile stones. In this case, therapy must be instituted without delay in order to prevent severe complications such as hemorrhagic pancreatitis, necrosis of the pancreas or biliary sepsis. According to the studies of Brunkhorst et al. (33-35, 38), patients with biliary pancreatitis presented with extremely high PCT concentrations (60.8±13.6 ng/ml, n = 13). Patients with pancreatitis of toxic etiology, e.g. alcohol abuse, presented with low PCT values (0.39±0.38 ng/ml, n = 19). In patients with negative ERCP (endoscopic retrograde cholangiography) findings, PCT values were significantly lower than those with a diagnosis of biliary pancreatitis. There was no difference in levels of CRP, neopterin, IL-6 and bilirubin between these groups (Figure 4.6.2). PCT concentrations over 1 ng/ml on the day of hospital admission should therefore indicate obstruction of the biliary system. The authors recommend early antibiotic therapy and ERCP in patients with hyperprocalcitoninemia and acute pancreatitis unless the disease is due to cholangitis (35, 38).

The findings of Brunkhorst et al. are corroborated by the studies of Oezcueruemez-Porsch et al. (132) who did not observe increased PCT values in only mild pancreatitis following diagnostic ERCP without systemic or infectious complications but noted a significant rise in CRP, IL-6, IL-10, serum-amyloid A and IL-1RA levels. At this point it should also be noted that use of PCT in the differential diagnosis of biliary and toxic etiologies of pancreatitis is useful only in the early stages of the disease as other factors exert an increasing influence on PCT induction as the disease advances. Effective differential diagnosis assumes that no additional complications such as concomitant bacterial diseases or septic shock are present.

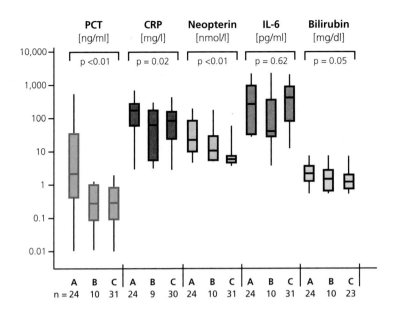

Figure 4.6.2

Box-plot diagram of PCT, neopterin, IL-6 and CRP values in patients with biliary (Group A) and non-biliary or toxic pancreatitis (Group C). Group B is a sub-group of Group A with negative findings on ERCP. Results are indicated as median (-), 25% and 75% percentiles (box) and minimum-maximum values. P = level of significance in the Mann-Whitney test between Groups A and C (n = No. of measurements) (according to 34).

4.7   ARDS (Acute Respiratory Distress Syndrome): bacterial and toxic etiology

ARDS (Acute Respiratory Distress Syndrome) is characterized by severe alterations of the lung structure. The characteristically altered X-ray pattern of the lung and refractory hypoxemia are typical sequelae of increased capillary permeability and of the profound cellular alterations of the lung structure.

The etiology can range from infectious and bacterial diseases to non-bacterial or toxic causes such as alcohol-induced delirium, severe side effects of medication (39), embolism and autoimmune disorders. Treatment varies depending on the etiology and should always rule out the underlying noxious substances. It is often difficult to recognise the etiology of ARDS under clinical conditions.

The differential diagnosis of ARDS

If the etiology of ARDS cannot be sufficiently determined, determination of PCT levels may prove a useful diagnostic tool. Brunkhorst *et al.* (37) reported PCT levels of substantially over 5 ng/ml in patients with ARDS of bacterial etiology. Toxin-induced ARDS was, however, characterized by only slightly elevated PCT concentrations (<3 ng/ml, $p = 0.0003$, MWU test). Discrimination between groups was not feasible with IL-6 and CRP ($p = 0.1831$ and 1.0 respectively) since these parameters were clearly increased by non-specific inflammation in both diagnostic groups. Only neopterin levels allowed differentiation between infectious and non-infectious etiologies, albeit with less significance (Figures 4.7.1 to 4.7.3).

ARDS is often triggered secondary to sepsis, pneumonia, multiple trauma or in the course of multiple organ dysfunction syndrome. Since PCT levels are generally increased due to these diseases, a more accurate differentiation between toxic and non-toxic etiologies of ARDS will prove impossible in many cases.

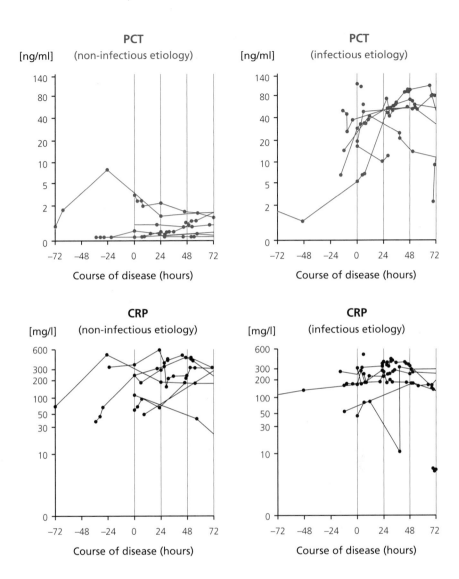

Figure 4.7.1

ARDS of infectious and non-infectious etiology: Clearly differentiated PCT values are a useful diagnostic and therapeutic tool. This differentiation is not feasible with CRP. Disease onset: t = 0, time in hours (37).

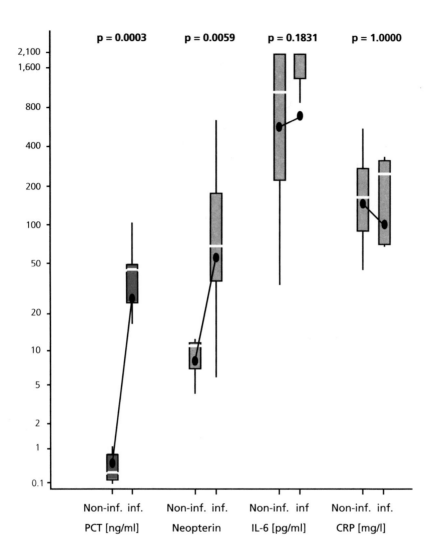

Figure 4.7.2

Box-plot of maximum concentrations of PCT, neopterin, IL-6 and CRP within the first 24 hours after onset of ARDS. Groups are categorized by infectious and non-infectious etiology of the disease. Results are indicated as median (-), mean (.), standard error of the mean (SEM) (box) and maximum-minimum values (37).

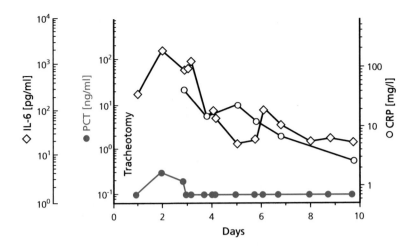

Figure 4.7.3

Case report of non-infectious ARDS after exposure to enalapril with edema of the glottis and ARDS. IL-6, CRP and PCT values are illustrated over a course of 10 days. PCT values did not exceed the normal range of 0.5 ng/ml at any time (39).

Pneumonia and hyperprocalcitoninemia

PCT is induced in acute bacterial pneumonia provided that systemic inflammation is present. Since pneumonia is generally an organ-
related infection, PCT values are usually low even in the presence
of marked clinical symptoms or X-ray findings (Figures 4.1.1 and
4.3.4c) (68, 88).

Slight PCT induction in pneumonia

PCT induction is generally slight in isolated pneumonia due to the
organ-related nature of the infection. Whether or not this slight
rise in PCT can be detected clinically will depend on the accompanying circumstances, *i.e.* the patient's previous medical history or
the corresponding patient population, *e.g.* post-surgical patients.
Only slight PCT induction may therefore be observed with pneumonia in the case of acute community-acquired pneumonia in an
otherwise healthy subject. In ICU patients, however, the rise in PCT
levels is often eclipsed by other influential factors since numerous
stimuli affect these patients and can induce PCT. Therefore, PCT
cannot be routinely used to diagnose pneumonia in hospitalized
patients. Diagnosis should not be the primary aim of PCT determination in these patients since organ-related or local infections do
not induce PCT and pneumonia can be accurately diagnosed by
other means. PCT concentrations are high only in cases of an infectious complication characterized by systemic inflammation (sepsis,
septic shock) (Figure 4.1.1).

PCT as an indicator of the risk of lung failure?

PCT is an early indicator of a high risk of subsequent pulmonary
dysfunction and other risks. This has been demonstrated in several studies involving multiple trauma patients and patients having
undergone major surgery.

According to studies conducted by Hensel *et al.* (76), increased PCT
values observed after cardiac surgery were frequently correlated

with acute lung failure. In cases of multiple trauma patients, patients who went on to develop lung complications displayed significantly higher PCT values within the first 12 to 24 hours of the accident compared with those patients who developed no such complications over the course of the first 6 days (see chapter 4.4).

Community-acquired pneumonia

Nylen et al. (120) reported high immunoreactive calcitonin (iCT) (1.0 ± 0.4 ng/ml iCT, normal population 0.03 ng/ml iCT) in 12 patients with isolated acute community-acquired pneumonia. In patients with positive bacterial cultures, the values were higher than those observed with negative bacterial findings (6 patients each, 1.8 ± 0.7 ng/ml and 0.2 ± 0.1 ng/ml iCT respectively).

Gramm et al. (68) also reported slightly elevated PCT concentrations in acute community-acquired pneumonia. Values of 0.2 ng/ml PCT were detected in 149 patients (median, range: 0.1–6.7 ng/ml). By way of comparison, values of 3 ng/ml (1.1–35.3 ng/ml) and 31.8 ng/ml (range: 0.5–5420 ng/ml) were recorded in peritonitis and sepsis respectively.

De Werra et al. (49) described similar findings in patients with severe community-acquired pneumonia. Values of 2.4 ± 3.7 ng/ml PCT (mean ± SD) were recorded compared with 96 ± 181 ng/ml in septic shock. In this study, "severe" indicated the presence of at least two additional symptoms taken from the following list in addition to radiological diagnosis: fever, leukocytosis, expectoration or cough.

Hospital-acquired pneumonias

In patients with hospital-acquired pneumonias, Cheval failed to observe a significant difference between plasma PCT concentrations in 29 ICU patients with confirmed pneumonia versus no pneumonia (6.9 ± 12 ng/ml and 3.8 ± 6 ng/ml PCT, p = 0.98). Similarly, the PCT measured in bronchioalveolar lavage fluid did not differ between the two groups (p = 1).

Aspiration pneumonia

Hyperprocalcitoninemia is frequently observed in aspiration pneumonia (120, 122) (own studies). Values fall within a few days if there are no complications (Figures 4.8.1 and 4.8.2).

Inhalation trauma

Increased PCT values of varying degree were observed following inhalation trauma (see chapter 4.15).

Chronic lung diseases

Individual cases of slightly raised PCT values have also been observed in otherwise healthy patients with chronic lung diseases. Becker *et al.* (11) detected slightly increased PCT concentrations in heavy smokers and patients with chronic obstructive bronchitis. These values were, however, only marginally above those of a normal healthy population. Chronic inflammation and bacterial superinfection with diminished lung clearance attributable to cigarette smoke or chronic obstructive bronchitis as well as the hyperplasia of neuroendocrine cells described as a sequella of cigarette smoke could account for this finding (160). Slightly increased PCT values also occur as a delayed reaction to inhalation trauma (118).

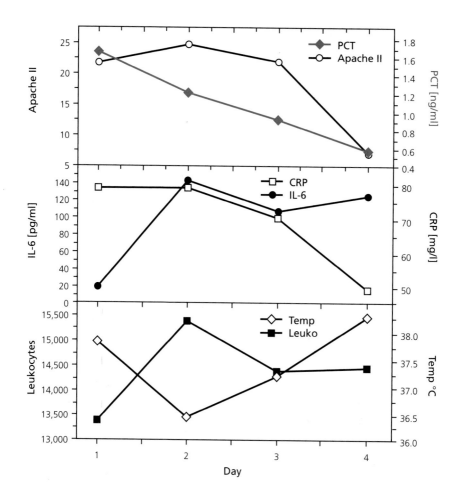

Figure 4.8.1

Case illustration: Complication-free course following massive aspiration confirmed by bronchoscopy. PCT values fell rapidly during antibiotic therapy in line with clinical improvement (T. Palmaers, M. Meisner).

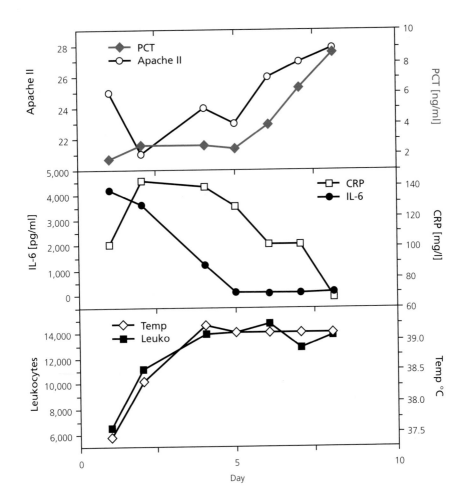

Figure 4.8.2

Case illustration: 17 year-old male patient with fulminating course of aspiration pneumonia and ARDS. Clinical data indicate on-going exacerbation of the pulmonary situation. Initial PCT values were only slightly raised but increased rapidly starting from the 6th day after disease onset. In view of the increasing number of symptoms, extracorporeal oxygenation was administered on the 8th day (T. Palmaers, M. Meisner).

4.9   Autoimmune disorders, chronic non-bacterial inflammation and neoplastic disorders

Chronic, non-bacterial inflammation does not induce PCT. Also autoimmune disorders and other systemic disorders with occasionally severe symptoms of inflammation such as vasculitis or systemic lupus erythematosus do not normally increase plasma PCT concentrations. Similarly, other non-infectious diseases and neoplastic diseases do not induce PCT.

Autoimmune disorders and systemic disorders

Eberhard et al. (50) examined 53 patients with autoimmune disorders. 18 of these patients presented with systemic lupus erythematosus and 35 patients with systemic anticytoplasmic antibody-related vasculitis (M. Wegener and microscopic polyangitis). PCT levels of less than 0.5 ng/ml were detected in 99% of plasma samples collected from these patients whereas neopterin, IL-6 and CRP concentrations in patients with active, underlying disease were raised to the pathological range (Figure 4.9.1). Infections were detected in 11 patients with PCT values averaging 1.93 ± 1.19 ng/ml (Figure 4.9.2).

Another group (Stroehmann et al.) reported on PCT values in 83 patients presenting with various inflammatory rheumatic disorders including reactive arthritis, systemic lupus erythematosus, scleroderma, myositis, vasculitis and fibromyalgia. Although many of the patients presented with highly active disease with marked symptoms of inflammation and increased proinflammatory cytokines, plasma PCT concentrations were still within the normal range. Schwenger et al. reached the same conclusion in a study involving 25 patients with systemic lupus erythematosus and 27 patients with rheumatoid arthritis (151).

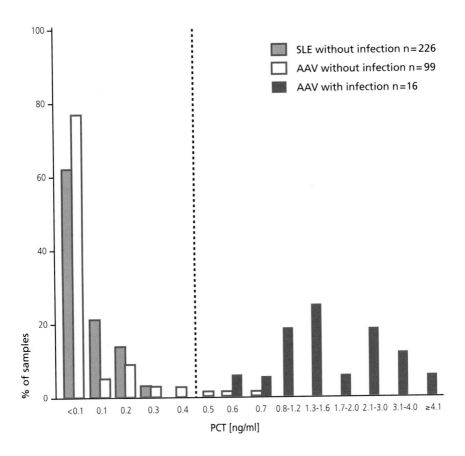

Figure 4.9.1

Distribution of the mean values of PCT in serum samples collected from patients with systemic lupus erythematosus (SLE, 18 patients, all without infection) and with anti-neutrophil antibody-related vasculitis (AAV, 35 patients) with and without bacterial infection (systemic infection, 16 patients). The values were measured in the early stages of infection. The dotted line indicates the normal range of PCT values (50).

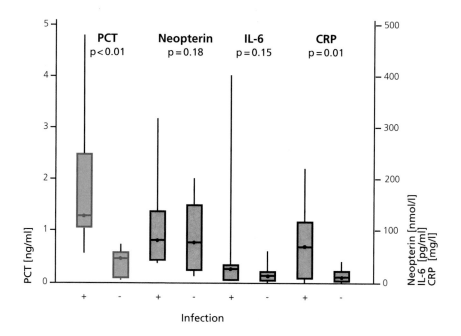

Figure 4.9.2

PCT, neopterin, IL-6 and CRP serum concentrations in 11 patients with antibody-related vasculitis during 16 bouts of systemic infection compared with an infection-free interval 4–6 weeks before or after corresponding treatment (p, Wilcoxon test) (50).

Slightly increased PCT values can be measured in individual cases in patients presenting with active Wegener's granulomatosis. Ninety-five per cent (95%) of the PCT values were below 0.89 ng/ml in the absence of infection (151). Moosig et al. (115) reported PCT values above the normal range of 0.5 ng/ml in 3 out of 26 patients with this disease. These three patients presented with values ranging from 0.8 to 3.3 ng/ml. Schwenger et al. (151) therefore recommend PCT values <1.0 ng/ml as the cut-off point for the diagnosis of invasive infections accompanying this disease.

Other non-infectious disorders

Angio-edema
Normal PCT values were reported in a patient with angio-edema (39).

Adrenocortical failure
Impaired adrenocortical function can be associated with symptoms resembling sepsis. In such cases, a diagnosis of septic shock in the absence of elevated PCT concentrations could be challenged, and the diagnosis of adrenocortical failure was confirmed (75).

Rectocolitis
C. Bohoun (27) examined 17 patients with rectocolitis. All the patients presented with PCT values below 1 ng/ml. Leukocytosis and a slight fever were observed in three patients with values between 0.5 ng/ml and 1 ng/ml. In most cases, elevated PCT values in disorders of non-bacterially induced inflammation therefore indicate a bacterial infection or an additional infectious, feverish condition but not an acute episode of an autoimmune disorder.

Neoplastic disorders and malignancies

Patients with neoplasia or malignant tumours usually have normal or only slightly increased PCT concentrations. In these patients increased PCT levels are found only if systemic inflammation is present.

Bohoun *et al.* (27) reported on 30 patients with myeloma and Morbus Waldenström. 24 of these patients had PCT concentrations below 0.1 ng/ml and 6 patients had PCT levels between 0.1 and 1 ng/ml. Out of 37 patients with prostate cancer, 35 had normal PCT values. 2 patients with severe urogenital infections presented with increased PCT levels. Brunkhorst *et al.* (F.M. Brunkhorst, personal communication) examined 10 patients with different malignant tumors including patients with bronchial carcinoma and lymphoma and likewise found only slightly elevated PCT values despite markedly increased neopterin concentrations.

Exceptions: increased PCT values in specific non-bacterial disorders

Tumour disorders

Individual tumours may synthesise peptides similar to calcitonin and calcitonin precursor proteins. This has been established for the following three types of tumour: increased serum PCT and calcitonin values have been detected in medullary C-cell carcinoma of the thyroid (MCT) (20, 71, 154). Increased immune reactivity to PCT, calcitonin precursor molecules and calcitonin can also be detected in small cell carcinoma of the lung and in bronchial carcinoma (10, 12, 13, 23, 24, 121).

COPD and chronic bronchitis

Minimally increased concentrations of calcitonin precursor molecules can be detected in patients presenting with chronic-obstructive lung disease and chronic bronchitis. Alternatively, the slight increase could be a late reaction to inhalation trauma (14, 19, 118).

Portal hypertension, liver cirrhosis (Child C stage)

Elevated PCT values were detected in portal hypertension and especially in decompensated portal hypertension (F.M. Brunkhorst, personal communication). The etiology of the disease is thus irrelevant. Increased bacterial translocation and endotoxin release from the intestine due to portal vein blockage are probably responsible for this observation. Significantly elevated PCT values have also been reported in patients with severe liver cirrhosis (Child C but not Child A or B).

Peritoneal dialysis

Slightly elevated basal PCT concentrations have also been detected in patients undergoing peritoneal dialysis.

4.10 PCT in the differential diagnosis of viral and bacterial infections

In disorders triggered solely by viral pathogens, the body reacts with only a slight increase in PCT values if at all. PCT can therefore be used for the differential diagnosis of viral versus bacterial infections provided that systemic inflammation accompanies the bacterial infection. Differential diagnosis is therefore significant in cases where a rapid decision between bacterial and non-bacterial etiology of the infection has therapeutic consequences. Gendrel *et al.* (61) could detect significant differences in PCT concentrations in establishing viral versus bacterial etiology in children with meningitis. In these cases, PCT was used as an early and sensitive indicator of bacterial-induced meningitis (see chapter 4.16) (26, 60, 62). Differential diagnosis of viral and bacterial infections is also relevant in immunodeficient or immunosuppressed patients, *i.e.* in transplantation medicine, in neutropenic patients and following chemotherapy.

The differential diagnosis of viral and bacterial meningitis

Markedly increased plasma PCT concentrations were detected in children presenting with acute bacterial as opposed to viral meningitis (61). The parameter can be used to confirm rapid diagnosis of bacterial versus viral meningitis. Comparison of PCT values with other inflammatory parameters in meningitis is presented in chapter 4.16.

HIV infection (AIDS)

Increased PCT values were not found even in the advanced stages of disease in HIV-positive patients (3, 63). In the presence of sepsis, however, PCT induction was observed, even in HIV infections. Secondary infections in the form of *Pneumocystis carinii*-induced pneumonia (PCP), cerebral toxoplasmosis, tuberculosis, viral infections or local bacterial or fungal infections do not trigger an increase in PCT concentrations in HIV-infected patients provided that these are organ-related or local infections without systemic inflammation (63).

Hepatitis B, CMV

PCT concentrations were within normal limits or only slightly above the normal range in cases of acute hepatitis B (F.M. Brunkhorst, personal communication) and CMV infections.

4.11 Fungal infections: *Candidiasis* and *Aspergillosis*

Elevated PCT values have been reported time and time again in systemic fungal infections (*Candidiasis, Aspergillosis*) (64, 88, 156, 158). There is, however, also evidence to suggest that PCT is not induced in these infections. Reference is made to case reports relating to four patients with *Aspergillosis* and *Candidiasis* in whom only minor PCT induction was observed (8, 79). In these cases, however, the severity of the systemic inflammation was not adequately documented. The absence of PCT induction due to a lack of systemic inflammation cannot, therefore, be ruled out. *C. albicans*-positive blood cultures were clinically correlated with sepsis in only one of these cases without corresponding induction of PCT.

Varying observations warrant further studies

Further observations are therefore required in order to confirm or rule out induction of PCT by fungal infections. Based on current data, PCT induction due to fungal infections cannot be confirmed at the present time. Elevation of PCT levels observed in many cases of *Candidiasis* and *Aspergillosis* may be based on the secondary effects of induction via bacterial translocation or accompanying sepsis.

4.12 Tropical diseases and malaria

Increased PCT concentrations have been reported in both uncomplicated and severe forms of malaria. The highest values are measured in the more severe forms of the disease. In response to therapy, serum concentrations quickly fall within a few days. These observations, initially reported by Davis *et al.* (47, 48) were corroborated in a study by Al-Nawas and Shah (4). 38 patients with suspected malaria presented with PCT values averaging 5.3 ng/ml in confirmed infection [standard error of the mean (SEM) 1.56, n = 17]. Patients in whom malaria infection was not confirmed presented with average values of 0.43 ng/ml PCT (SEM 0.64, n = 21) on the day of admission. The authors calculated 52% sensitivity and 86% specificity for the diagnosis of malaria with a cut-off value of 2 ng/ml for PCT. There was a correlation between plasma PCT levels and initial parasite density which was used as a marker of disease severity (78). Correlation of PCT with serum-bilirubin levels was indicative of liver damage in studies conducted by Davis et al (47).

Unknown induction mechanism in the case of malaria

PCT is obviously not a specific diagnostic tool for the detection of plasmodia. Elevated plasma PCT levels may reflect the marked systemic inflammatory reaction in malarial infection. PCT cannot, in any way, replace specific studies such as microscopic studies in droplets. Therapy must not be limited in any way because of lower PCT values.

Other tropical diseases: melioidosis

Melioidosis is another tropical disease in which very high PCT concentrations have been reported (152). This is not surprising since the disease is triggered by a bacterium of the group of pseudomonas, *Burkholderia pseudomallei*. Melioidosis can often become a fulminating, life-threatening disease if not treated in time. The symptoms of the disease are not always clear and range from slight, chronic discomfort, gastrointestinal symptoms and sudden fever to septicemia, pneumonia and abscess formation. Commencement of early antibiotic treatment is essential. Melioidosis is endemic in Southeast Asia and North Australia. There is also a good correlation between serum PCT concentrations and disease severity in cases of melioidosis (152). PCT is not a specific diagnostic tool for this disease but nevertheless sounds the alarm, thus indicating a severe, potentially life-threatening complication of infection due to systemic inflammation. Regardless of PCT levels, as in the case of malaria, specific individualized therapy must be instituted as soon as the diagnosis is confirmed either clinically or on the basis of laboratory tests.

4.13   Immunosuppression and leukopenia

Patients with an impaired response of the immune system are predisposed to infection. Impaired immunity can be triggered iatrogenically through immunosuppressants, after transplantation, by chemotherapy, irradiation or in the presence of malignant or viral diseases, especially HIV infection. Patients with an impaired immune response are highly predisposed to infections and will thus benefit from PCT determination. Studies to date have demonstrated that PCT is synthesized and released in response to appropriate stimuli in the face of immunosuppression and leukopenia.

Transplantation: immunosuppressants and corticosteroids

Immunosuppressants and corticosteroids are regularly used following organ transplantation. The response of PCT to bacterial infection remains unchanged with this medication. Many authors have reported PCT increase in systemic infections following liver, heart or kidney transplantation as well as after allogenic and autologous stem cell transplantation (52, 56, 57, 72, 89, 93, 155, 158, 170).

PCT and TNF-α induction is unchanged under high-dose steroid therapy whereas IL-6 synthesis is markedly suppressed (72, 155, 158).

Leukopenia

According to studies conducted by Al-Nawas (3) on PCT values in 122 patients with immune deficiency of varying etiology, no difference in PCT values was observed in these patients compared with non-immunosuppressed patients at the onset of infection (Day 0 to 2). During the subsequent course of the condition (Day 3 to 5), PCT levels were significantly lower in patients with an impaired immune system or presenting with neutropenia than in a septic control population with an intact immune system. In immunosuppressed patients, values were essentially within the normal range at this same time period (p = 0.02). A similar picture is observed if the leukocyte count is used as the criterion for immunosuppression. Patients with leukocyte counts below 4.5 /nl presented with plasma PCT levels on the 1st and 2nd day after onset of the induced event which were comparable to those observed in patients with normal leukocyte counts. Values in leukopenic patients were, however, distinctly lower after the 2nd day. In this study, the level of significance was not reached. The immune deficiency in patients in this study was caused by various underlying diseases: 20 patients presented with HIV-infection, 13 had acute myeloblastic or lymphoblastic leukemia and 7 patients had kidney or liver transplants while another 15 patients presented with other malignant disorders of the hematopoietic system.

Studies carried out by other authors confirm that PCT levels respond much the same way to fever and infections in neutropenic patients and non-neutropenic patients.

According to investigations conducted by Kou (86), PCT values are similar in both febrile, neutropenic patients (n = 25) and febrile non-neutropenic patients (n = 15) with underlying malignant hematological diseases. The values reported for non-neutropenic patients were slightly higher than those of neutropenic patients, albeit not to any significant degree.

Fleischhack et al. (56, 57) observed marked PCT induction in systemic infections, especially in the case of Gram-negative bacteremia (Table 4.13.1) in children presenting with neutropenia and underlying malignant disease. The authors concluded that PCT induction remained the same in this patient population.

Table 4.13.1

Diagnostic certainty of PCT and CRP in neutropenic patients for the diagnosis of Gram-negative bacteremia at the time of admission (57).

	PCT	CRP
Positive predictive value	100%	0%
Negative predictive value	94.9%	92.2%
Specificity	100%	100%
Sensitivity	45.4%	0%

Lestin *et al.* (93) published in-depth data on PCT induction in cytostatic-induced neutropenia. The studies were conducted in 112 patients with hematological disorders. PCT values rose significantly with confirmed infection in patients whose condition was characterized by neutropenia and fever whereas concentrations were within the normal range in patients with malignant hematological disorders but free from fever and infection. Compared with other parameters (CRP, IL-6, IL-1), PCT had a high sensitivity of 77% and specificity of 96% for the diagnosis of systemic infection in neutropenic patients presenting with a high temperature.

HIV

The immune system is known to be progressively damaged following HIV infection (AIDS). Whereas HIV infection does not induce PCT itself, the impaired immune system has no quantifiable effect on PCT induction secondary to severe bacterial infection (3, 63). High PCT concentrations were observed in patients with HIV infections and sepsis whereas values below 2.1 ng/ml were reported in various localized infections. Mean PCT values in clinically stable patients in all categories of the CDC classification were only slightly, albeit not significantly, higher (PCT 0.5 ± 0.37 ng/ml) than those observed in a normal population (63).

Neoplastic diseases

Neoplastic diseases can also affect the immune system. This applies in particular to malignant, hematological disorders. PCT synthesis is not adversely affected by the underlying disease in patients with infectious complications (56, 57, 93, 170). PCT synthesis is not diminished following myeloablative therapy and during chemotherapy for cytoreduction. It should be noted that certain types of solid tumours may synthesize and release PCT and other calcitonin precursor proteins paraneoplastically (see chapter 4.9).

In various malignant diseases, tumour tissue can be made to regress by chemotherapy or irradiation. Cytoreduction via various combinations of cytostatic agents constitutes first-line treatment. Cytoreducing therapy treats immune deficiency as an undesirable side effect due to the high proliferation of immunocompetent cells. This can also be a principal effect in bone marrow transplantation. Immune deficiency is generally associated with neutropenia and with a high risk of infection. The immediate treatment of bacterial infections with an antibiotic will have a considerable effect on patient prognosis (93). Neutropenic patients, however, often fail to present with the characteristic signs of infection: leukocytosis, left-shift and local signs of inflammation are generally only minor. Specific parameters such as fever or C-reactive protein as inflammatory markers are not sufficiently specific.

PCT induction under immunosuppression and neutropenia

PCT follows a similar pattern in both immunosuppressed and neutropenic patients to that observed in patients whose immune system is not compromised (see chapter 4.13). PCT induction can also occur in neutropenic patients with septic complications.

Chemotherapy in malignant hematological disorders

Lestin *et al.* (93) collected extensive data on PCT in patients with hematological disorders and cytostatic-induced neutropenia. A series of factors were established in addition to PCT and clinical data in 112 patients during the course of chemotherapy. PCT values prior to chemotherapy were within the normal range in patients without fever or signs of infection (median 0.1 ng/ml). Similarly, PCT levels did not vary from the known reference range of 0.5 ng/ml even in patients with cytostatic-induced neutropenia without fever or signs of infection. Although within this reference range, values were nevertheless significantly higher than those recorded in a control population.

145

Fever and neutropenia: elevated PCT values in systemic infection

PCT levels were significantly increased in patients presenting with neutropenia and fever with confirmed infection in the presence of systemic inflammation whereas no significant increase was observed in locally confined infections or in fever of unknown origin (FUO) (93). If the PCT concentration is considered in relation to the pathogens, comparatively high PCT concentrations were found with Gram-negative pathogens in particular whereas PCT induction in cases of fungal infections was very slight or even non-existent (Table 4.14.1).

Multivariance analysis confirmed very high specificity and a somewhat lower degree of sensitivity for PCT compared with other parameters (Table 4.14.2). By combining a highly sensitive inflammation marker (CRP or neopterin) with a highly specific marker (PCT), over 90% of patients were correctly assigned to the infection group. In the other patients, infection was ruled out, thus providing indirect confirmation of a non-specific, tumour-induced inflammatory reaction (93).

According to the studies of Fleischhack *et al.* (56, 57), significantly increased PCT values were also observed in neutropenic children following chemotherapy, especially in cases of Gram negative bacteremia.

Table 4.14.1

Procalcitonin levels in patients with neutropenia and a temperature <38°C (93). PCT induction was insignificant with local and fungal infections compared with a significant induction in the case of systemic infections due to Gram negative and Gram positive pathogens. FUO = fever of unknown origin.

PCT [ng/ml]	Fungi	Gram positive bacteria	Gram negative bacteria
Median	0.6	1.1	10.7
Mean	1.4	6.2	21.1
SD	2.2	12.1	26.9
No.	6	7	3

	FUO	Local infection	SIRS/sepsis
Median	0.4	0.8	2.4
Mean	0.6	8.9	3.7
SD	0.6	16.9	0.4
No.	8	10	6

Table 4.14.2

Diagnostic values of selected cytokines and hemostasis parameters in malignant hematological disorders (patients with neutropenia and fever). PPV = positive predictive value, NPV = negative predictive value (according to 93).

Parameter	Cut-off	Sensitivity	Specificity	PPV	NPV
PCT (ng/ml)	0.5	0.77	0.96	0.91	0.89
IL-6 (pg/ml)	50	0.73	0.83	0.67	0.86
CRP (mg/l)	5	1	0.12	0.37	1
IL-1 (pg/ml)	40	0.17	1	1	0.75
Neopterin (nmol/l)	10	0.92	0.57	0.5	0.93
D-dimers Fibrin equiv./ml	120	0.82	0.83	0.69	0.9

Bone marrow transplantation

The immune defence mechanisms of patients receiving high doses of chemotherapy or total body irradiation as therapy for neoplastic disease or for purposes of immunosuppression is severely impaired. In addition to the immunosuppressant effect, the epithelial barriers of the mucosa and gastrointestinal tract are also adversely affected. Severe neutropenia further increases the risk of infection. Close monitoring of these patients for signs of infection is essential in addition to exposure prophylaxis. In some cases, it is also very difficult to distinguish between a graft-versus-host reaction and endotoxemia. In view of the indications for use of PCT, the potential diagnostic utility of this parameter should be examined further in severe immune defects or hematopoietic stem cell transplantation (HSCT).

In patients undergoing bone marrow transplantation, marked induction of PCT was apparent in the neutropenic phase following HSCT in 4 out of 19 patients (autologous HSCT) (170). The values ranged from 16 to 59 ng/ml PCT. Two of these patients presented with septic shock. In allogenic HSCT, 8 out of 30 patients exhibited elevated PCT values with septic shock. Values of up to 226 ng/ml were detected in this instance. These studies show that PCT can be formed even after virtually complete destruction of the hematopoietic system. The extent to which a non-specific increase in PCT values occurs in this particular context and the degree of sensitivity and specificity of the PCT response to infections must be investigated in further studies.

4.15   Burns and inhalation injuries

Early research into the precursor molecules of calcitonin demonstrated that immune-reactive calcitonin levels including PCT were known to markedly increase a few hours after burns involving inhalation injury (124). Initially high values were correlated with increased mortality. The correlation between premature deaths and inhalation injury was particularly high. By means of HPLC analysis, the authors confirmed that calcitonin measurements detected not only the hormone, calcitonin, but mainly the precursor molecules of calcitonin and fragments thereof, *i.e.* procalcitonin (119). A correlation with bacterial infections such as those described by Assicot *et al.* (1993) (7) was not, however, mentioned. The authors assumed that neuroendocrine cells of the bronchial epithelium (19) were responsible for the increased levels of calcitonin molecules. Hyperplasia and release of calcitonin precursor proteins are triggered by cigarette smoke in neuroendocrine cells (160).

Correlation with mortality levels and the extent of burns

The study carried out by Carsin *et al.* (43) was designed as a follow-up study in which PCT rather than immune-reactive calcitonin was measured in patients with burns in order to confirm the results obtained by O'Neill *et al.* in 1992 with immuno-reactive calcium (124). A series of interesting results was obtained in this study. At the time of patient admission, both PCT and IL-6 were actually prognostic factors for mortality. A median PCT value of 3.4 ng/ml (0.75–18.7 ng/ml, 25/75 percentile n = 21) was recorded in survivors compared with 7.0 ng/ml (25/75 percentile 2.1–44.1 ng/ml, n = 11) in fatal outcomes. The clinical Unit Burn Standard (UBS = percentage of body surface burned + 3-fold body surface with 3rd degree burns) is, however, far more reliable in terms of prognostic value. In this study, PCT values were not correlated with inhalation injury but with the extent of severe burns (>30% of the body surface).

According to studies conducted by D. von Heimburg *et al.* (163, 164), peak PCT values measured during the course of burns were correlated with the extent of the injured area (TBSA). This was not the case however with initial PCT values (r = 0.73, p <0.05, n = 27) (164). Plasma PCT levels were raised even on hospital admission. An average value of 2.1 ng/ml PCT was observed with 51% surface burns.

Early induction of PCT with burns

PCT is induced within 6 hours of the initial event in the case of burns. Bacterial infection is not present at this time because a fresh burn is sterile. Carsin *et al.* (43) measured plasma-endotoxin levels and TNF-α levels in their study to investigate the possible causes of PCT induction in burned patients. Neither parameter could be detected initially at the time when PCT is induced. Endotoxin was detected in very low concentrations in the plasma no earlier than 12 hours after the burn (Figure 4.15.1). These findings suggest that PCT can be induced by factors other than bacterial endotoxins, bacterial translocation or TNF-α after a burn. PCT correlates with serum-lactate concentrations which indicate the extent of tissue damage (hypoxia). PCT may therefore indicate the extent of tissue damage in burn patients since peak values are consistent with the UBS score within the first 24 hours. This is also the case for IL-6— another reliable marker of burn severity (161).

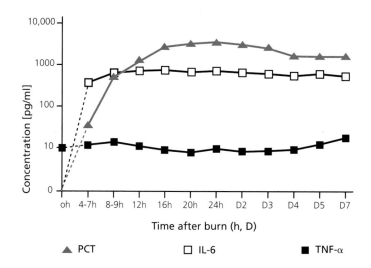

Figure 4.15.1

Time course of PCT, IL-6 and TNF-α serum concentrations in 40 patients with burn injury (mean values). Significant concentrations of endotoxin could only be detected 12 and 16 hours post-trauma (p <0.005 and 0.001, concentration 0 to a max. of 0.2 EU/ml. 1 EU is equivalent to 100 pg E. coli 0111: B4-1.2 endotoxin). h = hours, D = days after the onset of injury (43).

4.16   New-born infants and young children: Normal range, sepsis and meningitis

Rapid diagnosis and treatment of systemic bacterial infections is essential in neonates and infants. Since these young patients do not often present with specific symptoms, the clinical diagnosis must be supported by laboratory chemical and microbial results. Determination of PCT has proven to be an early and specific indicator of infection and sepsis in both neonates and young children.

Key topics and indications for the determination of PCT in neonates and young children are discussed in the following chapter.

PCT in neonates: reference range

PCT values are physiologically increased during the first few days of life so that a different reference range applies to premature and newborn infants (Table 4.16.1). The reference range for the first two days of life changes within a few hours (Figure 4.16.1) (45). The adult reference range applies three days after birth.

Table 4.16.1

The normal range of PCT values in neonates include 95% of all the measurements investigated in 83 healthy newborn infants according to age (hours) (45).

Normal range (including 95% of all measurements)			
Age in hours	PCT [ng/ml]	Age in hours	PCT [ng/ml]
0 – 6	2	30 – 36	15
6 – 12	8	36 – 42	8
12 – 18	15	42 – 48	2
18 – 30	21		

Studies confirmed that PCT levels can be raised in newborn infants without an accompanying infection (26, 114). Chiesa *et al.* (45) measured PCT levels in 83 healthy newborn infants and produced a 95% reference range (Figure 4.16.1). Peak values ranging from 0.1 to 21 ng/ml were reached on the first day after birth (median of 2 ng/ml). A marked fall in values was evident after 48 hours with a normal range of less than 2 ng/ml. PCT values of newborn infants with non-specific clinical signs and no evidence of infection were not different from those of normal newborn infants in terms of PCT values.

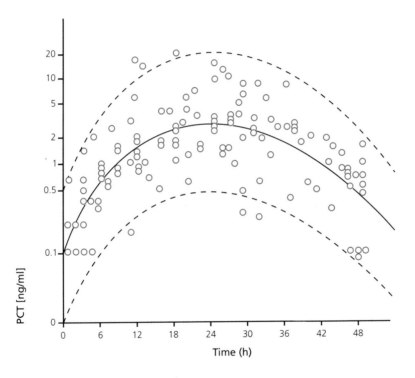

Figure 4.16.1

95% reference range of PCT in newborn infants (n = 83) in the first 48 hours after birth. Individual measurements are illustrated. The unbroken line characterizes the geometric mean and the dotted lines the 95% reference range (45).

Sepsis in neonates

Various authors have reported that PCT is an important marker for the early diagnosis of sepsis in neonates (45, 60, 62, 90, 114). The diagnostic sensitivity and specificity of PCT in the diagnosis of this condition can be as high as 100% (Table 4.16.2) (45). The unique reference range must, however, be observed in the first two days of life (Figures 4.16.1 and 4.16.2). PCT values in infected neonates clearly exceed this reference range (Figure 4.16.2) (45). This applies both to the early onset of sepsis within the first 48 hours of birth as well as to sepsis of later onset (in infants with an average age of 14 days). In both cases, the initial PCT values are significantly above the age-specific reference range.

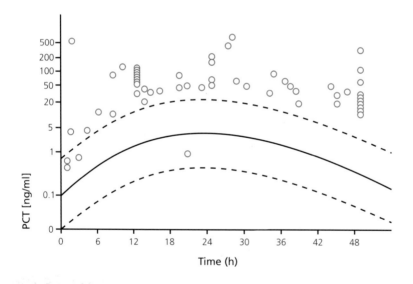

Figure 4.16.2

Procalcitonin values in neonates presenting with symptoms of infection within the first 48 hours of birth. Individual measurements are displayed. The unbroken line refers to the geometric mean while the dotted lines refer to the 95% reference range in the non-infected normal population (45).

Table 4.16.2

The diagnostic sensitivity and specificity of PCT determination in sepsis in neonates (45).

Infants aged 0–48 hours		Infants aged 3–30 days	
Early-onset sepsis		Late-onset sepsis	
Sensitivity	Specificity	Sensitivity	Specificity
92.6 %	97.5 %	100 %	100 %

PCT reacts more rapidly to an inflammatory stimulus than CRP. PCT values both rise and fall more rapidly than corresponding CRP levels (114). Sensitivity and specificity are considerably higher for PCT than CRP for the diagnosis of an infection and can be as high as 100% (Table 4.16.2). This is due in part to the fact that CRP reacts with a slower kinetic profile than PCT during the first 12 to 24 hours after the onset of an infection.

Monneret et al. (114) measured PCT levels in infection-free neonates and compared these with levels recorded in newborn infants presenting with maternofetal infections (n = 25) or secondary infections (n = 14). PCT levels were increased on the first day after birth even in neonates without infection (mean 3.82 ng/ml). Values were considerably higher in the case of maternofetal or secondary infections (162 ± 32 ng/ml and 75 ± 24 ng/ml respectively). On average, PCT increased in response to an infection or sepsis one day earlier than CRP. PCT levels also fell more rapidly after an infection compared with corresponding CRP values. This is illustrated by the case report of a male infant presenting with S. epidermidis infection in Figure 4.16.3 (114).

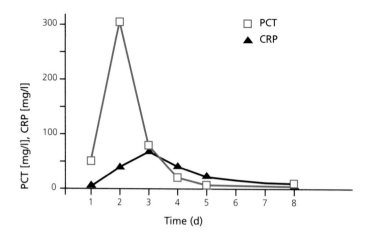

Figure 4.16.3

Time course of PCT and CRP values in a newborn infant presenting with S. epidermidis infection (114). Note the 24-hour interval in the peak values of both parameters and the comparatively rapid fall in PCT values.

PCT as a parameter for the early recognition of sepsis and severe bacterial infections in young children

As in adults, septic infections are also associated with elevated PCT values in young children. In this age group, PCT correlates with the activity of the inflammatory reaction and increases in response to an infection with systemic inflammation. Plasma PCT levels are not increased significantly by local infections or existing underlying diseases such as malignancies, allergies or autoimmune disorders.

Studies conducted by Assicot (7) and Gendrel (60) impressively confirm the fact that PCT is induced in children only with severe infections complicated by systemic inflammation, as opposed to viral infections, locally confined infections or superficial bacterial colonization. The results obtained by Gendrel are illustrated in Figure 4.16.4. No reliable discrimination between the groups could be made on the basis of CRP. High PCT values were found only in cases of sepsis.

The differential diagnosis of bacterial and viral infections in children

PCT discriminates between bacterial and viral infection with a high degree of sensitivity and specificity provided that symptoms of systemic inflammation are present (61, 62, 75). Even small quantities of bacterial toxins induce PCT synthesis. This accounts for the high PCT levels observed in bacterial infections with systemic inflammation. Synthesis is not, however, triggered in viral infections (Table 4.16.3).

Table 4.16.3

Procalcitonin values (mean, range) in children (aged 1 month to 12 years) with localized and systemic bacterial infections and viral infections (62).

	n	Mean (ng/ml PCT)
Systemic bacterial infection	30	29.7
Localized infection	20	1.7 (0.1–4.9)
Viral infection	70	0.28 (0.0–1.5)

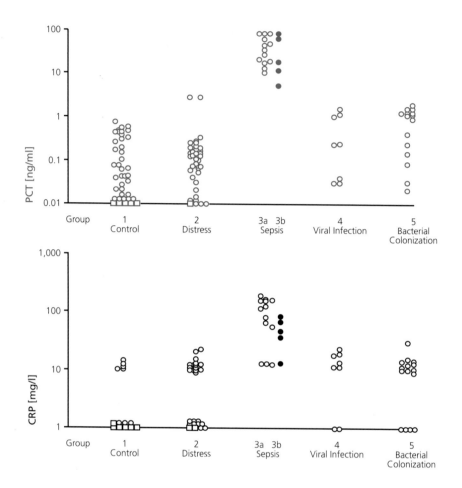

Figure 4.16.4

A comparison of CRP and PCT levels in 177 neonates. The individual values confirm the higher sensitivity and lower specificity of CRP in patients with systemic bacterial infections (60).

Group distribution: control group (n = 86): normal neonates; distress (n = 50): clinically suspect newborn infants with no signs of infection; sepsis (n = 13): clinical symptoms of sepsis and positive blood culture or CSF findings. Viral infections (n = 8): negative bacterial cultures, positive viral detection; bacterial colonization (n = 15): neonates with bacterial contamination of the skin during birth with no evidence of systemic infections. Normal range of PCT values: <0.5 ng/ml.

PCT values allow a more sensitive and specific discrimination of bacterial versus viral infections compared to CRP and other parameters. Significantly higher PCT values were observed in pediatric patients with bacterial as opposed to viral infections (Table 4.16.3). These observations were made primarily in patients presenting with meningitis (26, 60–62). PCT is therefore an important and useful parameter for the diagnosis of septic infection in both newborn infants and young children.

Additional studies of viral and bacterial infections in children

Gendrel *et al.* (62) reported on 70 children with confirmed severe viral infections and an average PCT value of 0.28 ng/ml. CRP levels were above 30 mg/ml in 11 out of 47 patients, and IL-6 concentrations were above 100 ng/ml in 9 out of 47 patients. 20 children with locally confined infections or negative blood cultures presented with an average PCT value of 1.7 ng/ml (mean, range: 0.1–4.97 ng/ml). An average value of 29.7 ng/ml was recorded in invasive bacterial infections. CRP values in the latter patients were below 30 µg/ml in 5 out of 30 children and IL-6 levels of less than 100 ng/ml were reported in 13 patients.

Comparison of acute viral versus bacterial meningitis

Tests to determine the protein and cell content of the CSF in some cases fail to rapidly differentiate between viral and bacterial meningitis in children. Many of the inflammatory parameters typical of both conditions cannot be adequately discriminated. Elevated plasma PCT values are detected only in acute bacterial meningitis (61). In viral meningitis PCT values lie within the normal range (Table 4.16.4).

Gendrel *et al.* (61) examined peripheral plasma PCT and CRP levels together with the cell and protein content of the CSF in 59 patients (aged >1 month). Increased PCT levels were observed in all children with bacterial meningitis while low values were observed in cases of viral meningitis (Table 4.16.4). CRP levels and CSF findings indicated significant overlapping in both groups.

The Bienvenu group in Lyon presented data on serum PCT levels in viral and bacterial infections (26). PCT values of >1 ng/ml were reported in 15 patients with bacterial meningitis compared with levels of <0.4 ng/ml in 12 patients with viral meningitis.

Table 4.16.4

Serum PCT and CRP values and the cell count and protein content of CSF in children presenting with acute bacterial meningitis or viral meningitis. The values are expressed as the mean ± SEM together with the range of values (61).

	Bacterial meningitis (n = 18)		Viral meningitis (n = 41)	
PCT ng/ml	54.5 ±	35.1 (4.8–110)	0.32 ±	0.35 (0–1.7)
CRP µg/ml	144.1 ±	69.1 (28–311)	14.8 ±	14.1 (0–48)
CSF-cell count/µl	5,156 ±4,336	(250–17,500)	390 ± 648	(20–3,200)
CSF-protein g/l	2.3 ±	1.2 (0.4–4.7)	0.62 ±	0.47 (20–3,200)

Similar data on bacterial meningitis and viral encephalitis were also published by Hatherill et al. (75).

PCT is thus an important parameter for the differential diagnosis of viral and bacterial forms of meningitis and can provide rapid information on bacterial-induced severe inflammation. The systemic-inflammatory reaction has not been quantified (by means of a score) in studies published to date. It is therefore impossible, at the present time, to assess the extent to which PCT values are influenced by the various degrees of systemic inflammation in these disorders.

In this context it should be noted that treatment of meningitis or of another infectious disorder of unknown etiology should never be omitted on the basis of low PCT values if other signs or the suspected clinical diagnosis suggest bacterial infection. PCT induction may not occur due to the local nature of an infection. Antibiotic treatment nevertheless may be mandatory to prevent the development of systemic inflammation and progression to an advanced stage of infection.

Local bacterial infection without PCT induction can also occur in adults. No rise in PCT values was observed in a patient with ventriculitis following neurosurgery as the infection is not accompanied by the symptoms of systemic inflammation (own observation).

A comparison of PCT and CRP levels in neonates and young children

C-reactive protein (CRP) has proved to be an early, sensitive indicator of infection in young children and neonates. CRP is an acute-phase protein that, in comparison with PCT, reacts to relatively minor infections. CRP can be induced to quite a substantial degree by non-specific events such as surgery (103) or by viral infections. The kinetic profile of CRP is also slower than that of PCT.

Compared to PCT, this acute-phase protein is therefore less suitable for the reliable assessment of the severity of an infection or related complication on the basis of systemic inflammation. CRP is a far more non-specific parameter than PCT for the diagnosis of severe bacterial infection or sepsis. PCT is not induced by localized and minor bacterial infections unless such infections are accompanied by a generalized systemic inflammation in addition to infection (45, 60, 114). The extent and significance of a severe infection can therefore be determined in both newborn infants and young children by means of PCT. In this respect, PCT is distinct from CRP as a parameter for the diagnosis of bacterial infections.

PCT reacts with more rapid kinetics at the beginning and end of an infection than CRP. Whereas an increase in PCT levels can be observed within the first 2–3 hours after an acute event and peak after as little as 12 to 24 hours, CRP values often only reach the pathological range after the same length of time. Even when the infection is regressing, CRP values often take several days to react and therefore take longer to fall than PCT (Figures 4.16.3 and 2.6.1).

5 Laboratory issues*

5.1 The laboratory determination of PCT: ILMA

The measurement of PCT with LUMItest® PCT, an immunolumino-metric assay (ILMA) manufactured by B·R·A·H·M·S Diagnostica GmbH is easy and can be completed within 2 hours.

In LUMItest® PCT, two antigen-specific monoclonal antibodies that bind procalcitonin (the antigen) at two different binding sites (the calcitonin and the katacalcin segments) are present in excess. One of these antibodies is luminescence-labeled (tracer) whereas the other is adhered to the inner wall of the test tube (coated tube system) (see Figure).

During the course of incubation, both antibodies react with the procalcitonin molecules in the sample to form so-called "sandwich complexes" whereby the luminescence labeled antibody is bound to the surface of the tube. Once the reaction is completed, the excess tracer is completely removed from the tube with careful rinsing and discarded.

The amount of residual tracer bound to the test tube wall after rinsing is quantified by measuring the luminescence signal using a suitable luminometer and the LUMItest® Basiskit reagents. The intensity of the luminescence signal (Relative Light Units, RLU) is directly proportional to the PCT concentration in the sample. After a standard curve has been established using standards with known antigen concentrations (calibrated against recombinant intact human procalcitonin), the unknown PCT concentrations in patient sera or plasma samples can be quantified by comparison to the standard curve.

---

* The information presented in chapter 5 is taken from the instruction leaflet for the LUMItest® PCT produced by B·R·A·H·M·S Diagnostica GmbH.

An alternative option is to determine the unknown PCT concentrations in patient sera or plasma samples using a master curve. The lot-specific data required to construct the master curve is produced by B·R·A·H·M·S Diagnostica GmbH and is included with each kit.

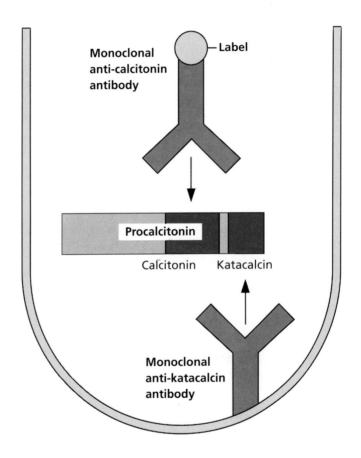

5.2   The LUMItest® PCT measuring kit

The LUMItest® PCT kit contains the reagents for 100 PCT determinations. The PCT values of 42 patients can be determined in duplicate using 6 standard preparations and 2 control samples.

The LUMItest® Basiskit which contains reagents needed to operate the luminometer is an essential accessory.

Contents of the reagent kit

This reagent kit is intended solely for *in-vitro* use. It contains sufficient quantities of the following components for 100 individual assays:

A   Coated tubes (test tubes)
Coated with anti-PCT antibodies (monoclonal, mouse)
2 sets of 50 tubes, **ready for use**

B   Tracer
Luminescence-labelled (acridinium derivate)
Anti-PCT antibody (monoclonal, mouse),
1 vial, lyophilized (freeze-dried), blue-coloured solution,
29 ml after reconstitution with buffer C

C   Buffer
For reconstituting tracer B,
1 vial containing 29 ml, **ready for use**

G   Zero serum (human serum)
For reconstituting the standards or calibrators and controls,
1 vial containing 4 ml, **ready for use**

W   Washing solution
Washing solution, concentrate,
2 bottles each containing 11 ml

S1, S2/K1, S3,   PCT standards
S4/K2, S5, S6
6 vials, **lyophilized**

Reconstitute each vial with 0.25 ml zero serum G prior to use.
Concentration ranges:
0.08 (def.); 0.3–0.7; 1.5–2.5; 16–24; 160–240; 400–600 ng/ml
For precise concentrations see leaflet enclosed. Standards S2/K1 and S4/K2 are used as calibrators K1 and K2 for the master curve.

Ko1, Ko2   PCT controls 1 and 2
2 vials, **lyophilized**
Reconstitute each vial with 0.25 ml zero serum G prior to use.
For concentrations see leaflet enclosed.

The following accessories are also required

- LUMItest® Basiskit (available on order from B·R·A·H·M·S Diagnostica GmbH)
- Micropipettes (20 µl, 250 µl) with disposable plastic tips
- Vibration mixer
- Horizontal rotator
- Dispenser (5 ml) for washing solution
- Distilled water
- Luminometer with two injectors

Contents of the LUMItest® Basiskit

The LUMItest® Basiskit from B·R·A·H·M·S Diagnostica GmbH contains sufficient quantities of the following components for 1,000 chemiluminescence measurements:

BR1 Basiskit reagent 1
0.5% H_2O_2 in 0.1 M HNO_3
3 bottles each containing 105 ml, **ready for use**

BR2 Basiskit reagent 2
0.25 M sodium hydroxide
3 bottles each containing 105 ml, **ready for use**

BK1 Basiskit control 1
2 vials, **lyophilized**; each containing 2 ml after reconstitution with distilled water

BK2 Basiskit control 2
2 vials, **lyophilized**; each containing 2 ml after reconstitution with distilled water

Stability and storage conditions

All reagents must be stored in kit packaging at a temperature of 4–8°C until required for use. Strictly comply with the expiry dates given on the kit packaging and reagent labels.

If less than 100 determinations are to be carried out, the following storage conditions shall apply for reconstituted reagents: *The reconstituted standards or calibrators and controls* must be stored at a temperature of −20°C (can be thawed ten times). The *reconstituted tracer* can be stored for 3 days at 4°C or should otherwise be stored at −20°C (can be thawed ten times).

The *diluted washing solution* can be stored for up to 4 weeks at a temperature of 4–8°C. Contaminated washing solution must not be used. This can be identified by turbidity or a pH of <6.

LUMItest® PCT incubation diagram

A. Standard curve

1. Number	test tubes	(a, b)	S1–S6	Ko1, Ko2	P1 etc.
2. Pipette	standards	µl	20	–	–
	controls	µl	–	20	–
	patient samples	µl	–	–	20
3. Pipette	tracer	µl	250	250	250
4. Incubate		1 h to 1 h 15 min at RT (18–25°C) on orbital shaker (170–300 rpm).			
5. Decant		Add 1 ml washing solution to each coated tube prior to decanting off the liquid.			
6. Wash		Add 1 ml washing solution to each coated tube four times and decant off the liquid. Turn the tubes upside down and allow them to drain on blotting paper for 5–10 min.			
7. Transfer		Place all coated tubes in luminometer.			
8. Measurement		Measure in luminometer with automatic injection of Basiskit reagents 1 and 2.			

B. Master curve

1. Number	test tubes		S2/K1, S4/K2	Ko1, Ko2	P1 etc.
2. Pipette	calibrators	µl	20	–	–
	controls	µl	–	20	–
	patient samples	µl	–	–	20
3. – 8.		See incubation diagram for standard curve.			

Specimen Handling

If samples are not analyzed within 4 hours after blood has been taken they must be stored at –20°C. Repeated freezing and thawing should be avoided.

Test Procedure

1.   **Preparations**

- Allow all kit components and patient samples to warm up to room temperature.
- Reconstitute tracer.
- Agitate all liquid reagents—including patient sera—gently before use (avoid foam formation).
- Number the coated tubes (preferentially using a, b for duplicates).
- Prepare washing solution: dilute 11 ml concentrate with distilled water to yield 550 ml. We strongly recommend to contact the manufacturer or distributor before using other washing solutions.
- Prepare the luminometer for use.

Note   In large series of tests, the reagents with identical batch numbers can be pooled.

2.   Pipette **20 µl PCT standards** of increasing concentrations into the tubes S1 a, b ... S6 a, b (resp. S2/K1, S4/K2 for the master curve). Pipette **20 µl of each control** into the tubes Ko1 a, b, Ko2 a, b, **and 20 µl of each serum sample or plasma** into the tubes P1 a, b etc. A new plastic micropipette tip should be used for each sample in order to avoid any carryover of PCT into subsequent samples.

Note   It is recommended not to change the sample matrix during a follow up analysis.

3.   Pipette **250 µl tracer** into all test tubes.

4. Mix the tubes for a short period of time on a sample mixer to ensure homogeneity of the liquid. Cover the test tubes with adhesive foil **and incubate them on a horizontal rotator (170–300 rpm) for 1 hour to 1 hour 15 minutes at room temperature (18–25°C)**.

Caution! **Protect the test tubes from light during incubation. Never expose test tubes to direct lighting.**

5. When the incubation is finished add 1 ml of the washing solution to each tube prior to decanting the liquid off completely.

When adding the washing solution, ensure that the upper section of the test tube wall is also completely wet with washing solution. This ensures that residual tracer that may be bound to the upper tube walls will also be removed.

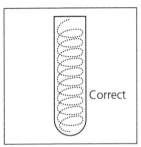

Correct

Correct addition
of washing solution

6. Subsequently, add **1 ml of the washing solution four times** to all test tubes (cf. no. 5) and decant off the liquid completely after each washing step.

After the **last rinsing step**, turn the tubes upside down and allow to drain for 5–10 minutes on clean blotting paper. Then tap the tubes gently on the blot-ting paper to remove any remaining liquid.

7. Place all tubes in the luminometer in the order defined by the measuring protocol.

8. Start luminescence measurement with automatic injection of 300 µl LUMItest® Basiskit reagents 1 and 2. **Recommended measuring time is 1 second per tube.**

Carefully follow the manufacturer's instructions. Improper handling of the reagents may falsify the test results. B·R·A·H·M·S Diagnostica GmbH is not liable for faulty test results arising from improper storage, use or handling.

Calculation of results

For computer-assisted analysis of LUMItest® PCT, a special program suitable for immuno-luminometric assays (spline algorithm is recommended for data evaluation) and which is compatible with the luminometer and computer hardware should be used.

Using the standard curve or the recalculated master curve resp., the measured luminescence signal values can then be used to directly determine the PCT concentration of the unknown samples in ng PCT/ml.

Example

Signal values (RLU = relative light units) obtained with an Auto-CliniLumat LB 952 (Laboratorium Prof. Berthold, Wildbad, D).

Test tube	RLU (a)	RLU (b)	RLU (MW)	ng PCT/ml
Standard S1	137	139	138	(def) 0.08
Standard S2	333	316	324	0.5
Standard S3	964	957	961	2.0
Standard S4	8,753	9,079	8,916	20
Standard S5	103,860	104,530	104,195	200
Standard S6	245,380	234,264	239,822	500
Patient sample P1	14,296	14,866	14,581	31.5

The signal values may vary depending on the measuring device used and are therefore given for information purposes only.

Standard curve

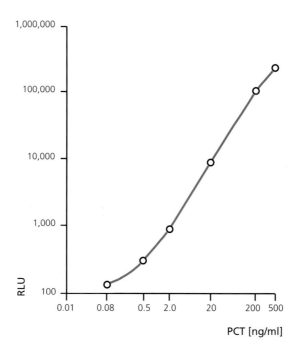

5.3   The master curve

PCT can also be determined using a "master curve". Lot-specific RLU data for each standard level are provided by B·R·A·H·M·S Diagnostica GmbH. The master curve is adjusted for each run using the two master curve calibrators supplied with the kit.

The master curve can be used to reduce the number of standards required to run the assay. This permits more time and cost efficient processing of test samples. The master curve calibrator values must be reentered in the luminometer when using a new lot.

Determination of PCT using a full standard curve is recommended for study purposes and with larger series of measurements. Variability in the values measured with the master curve are minor although concentrations can deviate by up to 20% under unfavorable conditions (incubation temperature of around 25°C).

See page 167 for the master curve incubation diagram.

5.4   Assay characteristics: precision, sensitivity, dilution and interference

Precision

The analytical assay sensitivity is approximately 0.1 ng/ml. The functional assay sensitivity (20% inter-assay variation coefficient) is approximately 0.3 ng/ml.

Dilution (with standard curve)

Sample	Dilution	Observed value [ng/ml]	Expected value [ng/ml]	Recovery (%)
1	Undiluted	140		
	1:2	77.0	70.0	110
	1:4	38.1	35.0	109
	1:8	19.1	17.5	109
	1:16	9.11	8.75	104
2	Undiluted	78.3		
	1:2	40.6	39.2	104
	1:4	19.9	19.6	102
	1:8	9.89	9.79	101
	1:16	4.9	4.89	100
3	Undiluted	60.5		
	1:2	33.2	30.3	110
	1:4	16.6	15.1	110
	1:8	8.36	7.56	111
	1:16	4.11	3.78	109
4	Undiluted	321		
	1:2	169	161	105
	1:4	82.0	80.3	102
	1:8	40.2	40.1	100
	1:16	19.5	20.1	97
5	Undiluted	90.1		
	1:2	48.1	45.1	107
	1:4	24.2	22.5	108
	1:8	11.7	11.3	104
	1:16	5.61	5.63	100

"High dose hook" effect (with standard curve)

The "high dose hook" effect is observed at PCT concentrations for 1,000 ng/ml and above.

Interferences to sequence analogous substances

Substance	Non-interfering concentrations
Calcitonin (human)	Up to 10 ng/ml
Katacalcin (human)	Up to 10 ng/ml
a-human CGRP*	Up to 10 000 ng/ml
b-human CGRP*	Up to 10 000 ng/ml

* Calcitonin Gene Related Peptide

Influence of medicaments

No influence on PCT measurements was recorded with antimicrobial chemotherapeutic agents, vasoactive drugs, analgesics, anticoagulants or diuretics. Drugs leading to a massive release of cytokines may increase the PCT level.

	Medicament	Cross reactivity (%)
Antimicrobial chemotherapeutic agents	Imipenem (Zienam®, MSD)*	$<1 \times 10^{-4}$
	Cefotaxim (Claforan®, Hoechst)*	$<4 \times 10^{-4}$
	Vancomycin (Vancomycin, Lederle)	$<1 \times 10^{-4}$
Vasoactive drugs	Dopamine (Dopamin, Fresenius)	$<1 \times 10^{-4}$
	Noradrenalin (Arterenol®, Hoechst)*	$<2 \times 10^{-4}$
	Dobutamin (Dobutamin Hexal)	$<5 \times 10^{-3}$
Others	Fentanyl (Fentanyl, Janssen)	$<1 \times 10^{-2}$
	Heparin	<100 IU/ml without effect
	Furosemide (Lasix®, Hoechst)*	$<1 \times 10^{-4}$

* Zienam® is a registered trademark of MSD, Claforan®, Arterenol® and Lasix® are registered trademarks of Hoechst.

5.5   Reference ranges

The following reference table can be drawn up from existing data relating PCT concentration to particular inflammatory conditions.

Patients	PCT [ng/ml]
Normal subjects	<0.5
Chronic inflammatory processes and autoimmune diseases	<0.5
Viral infections	<0.5
Mild to moderate localized bacterial infections	<0.5
SIRS, multiple trauma, burns	0.5–2
Severe bacterial infections, sepsis, multiple organ failure	>2 (often 10–100)

To assess the clinical course of an inflammatory response, the PCT concentration must be measured at least once a day during the course of the inflammatory process. An increase in PCT concentration indicates increased inflammatory activity, whereas a decrease in concentration points to a decrease in inflammatory activity which, in turn, indicates a more favourable prognosis.

It is recommended that each laboratory establishes and checks its own reference data using a representative patient collective. Therefore, the data given in the table above is for orientational purposes only.

6   The B·R·A·H·M·S PCT®-Q, a semi-quantitative rapid test*

6.1   Introduction

When PCT is used for differential diagnosis or to diagnose sepsis, the rapid availability of results is a distinct advantage. In many cases, however, acute determination of PCT is not feasible due to practical and organizational grounds, even if the doctor wishes to follow this approach. Additionally, not every hospital or facility where PCT can be used is equipped with a measuring device to determine PCT concentrations. As a result, PCT determination is often not implemented in an acute case, if at all, especially in situations where only a small number of samples are collected.

Thanks to the B·R·A·H·M·S PCT®-Q system, plasma PCT levels can now be determined anywhere, any time at a low cost. Using this particular test, semi-quantitative measurements are available within 30 minutes of collecting the plasma or serum sample and can be classified into four categories.

The test reading is sufficiently accurate for acute diagnosis and other diagnostic and therapeutic purposes. A distinction can be made between normal and elevated values (limit range 0.5 ng/ml) as well as between slightly (reference value 2 ng/ml) and markedly raised concentrations (over 10 ng/ml). Severe systemic inflammation secondary to infection (sepsis) can therefore be diagnosed with greater specificity compared with diseases presenting with only slightly elevated PCT values.

* The information given in Chapter 6 is taken from the instruction leaflet for B·R·A·H·M·S PCT®-Q produced by B·R·A·H·M·S Diagnostica GmbH.

6.2   Kit contents

The kit is for *in-vitro* use only. It contains the following components in sufficient quantities for 25 individual determinations:
- 25 individual test sets
- 25 reference cards
- 1 user leaflet

Each individual test set is sealed in protective packaging and contains:
- 1 individual test
- 1 disposable plastic pipette
- 1 dry bag

The B·R·A·H·M·S PCT®-Q must be stored in the unopened individual test packaging at **4–30°C**.

6.3 Measuring technique

The B·R·A·H·M·S PCT®-Q is an immunochromatografic test for the **semi-quantitative detection of PCT** (procalcitonin), which is used for diagnosing and controlling the treatment of severe, bacterial infection and sepsis. B·R·A·H·M·S PCT®-Q is a test system with an incubation period of only 30 minutes, which neither depends on apparatus, nor needs calibrating.

The test uses a monoclonal mouse anti-catacalcin antibody conjugated with colloidal gold (tracer) and a polyclonal sheep anti-calcitonin antibody (solid phase).

After the patient sample (serum or plasma) has been applied to the test strip, the tracer binds to the PCT in the sample and a marked antigen antibody complex forms. This complex moves by means of capillarity through the test system and, in the process, passes through the area containing the test band. Here, the marked antigen antibody complex binds to the fixed anti-calcitonin antibodies and forms a sandwich complex.

At a PCT concentration ≥0.5 ng/ml, this sandwich complex can be seen as a reddish band. The colour intensity of the band is directly proportional to the PCT concentration of the sample and is related to the following **PCT concentration ranges** with the help of a reference card:

<0.5 ng/ml   **≥0.5 ng/ml**   **≥2 ng/ml**   **≥10 ng/ml**

Non-bound tracer diffuses into the control band zone, where it is fixed and produces an intensely coloured red control band. The functional ability of the test system is checked by means of this control band.

Table

Possible interpretations of elevated PCT values and their diagnostic and therapeutic implications. The induction of PCT depends on the nature of the disorder and on the individual's clinical situation. The interpretations given here should thus be used for guidance only.

PCT concentration [ng/ml]	Interpretation	Options for further action (investigations, treatment)
<0.5	**Sepsis, severe sepsis or septic shock unlikely.** However, localized infections can not be excluded.	- Observe patient - Concentrate diagnostic investigations on clinical findings.
0.5–2	**Result needs further investigation, infection or sepsis possible.** **Severe sepsis or septic shock unlikely.**	- Search for the local focus of infection - Evaluate aetiologies for elevated PCT other than infection - Consider antibiotic therapy
2–10	**Bacterial infection complicated by systemic inflammation most likely.** **In some patients other causes are possible, e.g. major trauma or cardiogenic shock.**	- Intensify search for focus of infection - Evaluate aetiology of elevated PCT - Initiate specific and supportive therapy - Antibiotic therapy recommended, if indicated
>10	**Severe sepsis or septic shock most likely** **High risk to develope multiple organ dysfunction**	- Search for focus of infection - Initiate specific and supportive therapy - Intensive care strongly recommended

Definitions of sepsis, severe sepsis and septic shock according to ACCP/SCCM criteria (5).

Serial quantitative measurements of PCT every 24 hours are recommended.

6.4   Assay characteristics

Precision and accuracy

As a semi-quantitative test method, the B·R·A·H·M·S PCT®-Q correlates closely to the LUMItest® PCT with regard to the individual concentration ranges. Due to individual differences in the readings, differences between B·R·A·H·M·S PCT®-Q and LUMItest® PCT are possible, particularly in the proximity of the PCT concentrations symbolized by the reference band.

"High Dose Hook" effect

High PCT concentrations up to 4000 ng/ml have no affect on correct relating to the concentration ranges.

Interference

Haemoglobin values >5 g/dl (haemolytic) can restrict the reading accuracy and thus affect the test result. Therefore, severely haemolytic samples should not be measured with the B·R·A·H·M·S PCT®-Q.

Lipides or bilirubin have no effect on the measured result.

6.5   Test procedure

Note: Use a new individual test for each determination.

Prior to commencing with the test, bring the temperature of all components to room temperature.

Serum or plasma samples which are not used for the assay within 4 hours after taking the blood sample must be frozen and stored at −20°C. Repeated freezing and thawing is to be avoided.

1. Execution

The individual test packaging is not to be opened until immediately prior to measuring the samples.

Pipette **6 drops** using the enclosed dropper pipette into the round cavity of the B·R·A·H·M·S PCT®-Q. Fill pipette to at least the measuring line without any bubbles and hold slightly tilted when pipetting. Dispose of serum/plasma rests.

Note: Alternatively, a micropipette (200 µl) may also be used. Pipette **200 µl of serum/plasma** into the round cavity.

Incubate for 30 minutes at room temperature.

Document the time when the test was begun on the reference card.

2. Recording and assessment

After 30 minutes (max. 45 minutes), the PCT concentration range of the sample is determined.

Firstly, the validity of the test is checked with the help of the clearly visible **control band** (see ill. 1).

Illustration 1

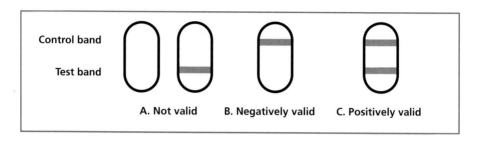

Control band

Test band

A. Not valid   B. Negatively valid   C. Positively valid

A. No band or only test band visible: tests, which show no control band are not valid and may not be evaluated.

B. Only control band visible: tests, which show only a control band are negatively valid. The PCT concentrations are <0.5 ng/ml.

C. Control and test band visible: tests, which show both a control band and a test band are positively valid.

The PCT concentration range is determined by **comparing the colour intensity of the test band with the colour blocks of the reference card** (see ill. 2).

Illustration 2

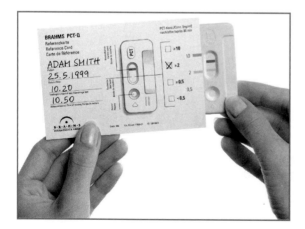

3. Documentation and archiving

To document the test result, the concentration range, which corresponds to the colour intensity of the test band, is marked with a cross on the reference card.

To archive the test result, the fully completed reference card can be stuck in the patient file (peel off the covering paper from the reverse of the reference card, to uncover adhesive tape).

Particular notes

1. The B·R·A·H·M·S PCT®-Q has 90–92% of diagnostic sensitivity and 92–98% of diagnostic specifity compared to LUMItest® PCT. Should, in the case of a positive result, a precise determination of the concentration be required from a clinical point of view, or an exact follow-up of the daily PCT concentrations be considered wise, we recommend that the samples be subsequently measured using the LUMItest® PCT.
2. A follow-up comparing a B·R·A·H·M·S PCT®-Q test visually with one from the previous day is not permitted, as the colour may change (from red to violet) within a few hours. It may also happen, that a test which is negative after 30 minutes may turn slightly in colour after a few hours. The result obtained after 30 minutes reading time is valid in this case.

Further information may be obtained from the Customer Service Department of B·R·A·H·M·S Diagnostica GmbH.

References

1. Abramowicz D, Schandene L, Goldmann M. Release of tumor necrosis factor, interleukin-2, and gamma-interferon in serum after injection of OKT3 monoclonal antibody in kidney transplant recipients. Transplantation 1989; 47:606-608.

2. Al-Nawas B, Krammer I, Shah PM. Procalcitonin in diagnosis of severe infections. Eur J Med Res 1996; 1:331-333.

3. Al-Nawas B, Shah PM. Procalcitonin in patients with and without immunosuppression and sepsis. Infection 1996; 24:434-436.

4. Al-Nawas B, Shah PM. Procalcitonin in acute malaria. Eur J Med Res 1997; 2:206-208.

5. Anonymous. American College of Chest Physicians/Society of Critical Care Medicine Consensus Conference: Definitions for sepsis and organ failure and guidelines for the use of innovative therapies in sepsis. Crit Care Med 1992; 20:864-874.

6. Ardaillou R, et al. Metabolic clearance rate of radioiodinated human calcitonin in man. J Clin Invest 1970; 49:2345-2352.

7. Assicot M, Gendrel D, Carsin H, Raymond J, Guilbaud J, Bohuon C. High serum procalcitonin concentrations in patients with sepsis and infection. Lancet 1993; 341:515-518.

8. Beaune G, Bienvenue C, Pondarre G, Monneret J, Bienvenue J, Souillet G. Serum procalcitonin rise is only slight in two cases of disseminated aspergillosis. Infection 1998; 26:168-169.

9. Becker KL, et al. Small cell lung carcinoma cell line express mRNA for calcitonin and alpha- and beta-calcitonin gene related peptide. Cancer Lett 1994; 81:19-25.

10. Becker KL, Gazdar AF. The pulmonary endocrine cell and the tumors to which it gives rise. Comparative Respiratory Tract Carcinogenesis, CRC Press, Bova Raton, FL 1983; 2:161-186.

11. Becker KL, Gazdar AF. The pathophysiology of pulmonary calcitonin. The endocrine lung in health and disease. Ed W B Saunders, Philadelphia 1984.

12. Becker KL, Gazdar AF. What can the biology of small cell cancer of the lung teach us about the endocrine lung? Biochem Pharmacol 1985; 34:155-159.

13. Becker KL, Gazdar AF, Carney DN, Snider RH, Moore CF, Silva OL. Calcitonin secretion by continuous cultures of small cell carcinoma of the lung: Incidence and immunoheterogeniety studies. Cancer Lett 1983; 18:179-185.

14. Becker KL, Nash DR, Silva OL, Snider RH, Moore CF. Increased serum and urinary calcitonin in pulmonary disease. Chest 1981; 79:211-216.

15. Becker KL, Nylen E, Thompson K. Preferantial hypersecretion of procalcitonin and its precursors in pneumonitis: a cytokine-induced phenomenony? Endotoxemia and Sepsis Congress 1995; (Abstract) Philadelphia, USA.

16. Becker KL, Nylen ES, Arifi AA, Thompson KA, Snider RH, Alzeer A. Effekt of classic heatstroke on serum procalcitonin. Crit Care Med 1997; 25:1362-1365.

17. Becker KL, Nylen ES, Cohen R, Snider RH. Calcitonin: structure, molecular biology, and actions. Princiles of Bone Biology, Academic Press Inc 1996; 1:471-494.

18. Becker KL, Nylen ES, Snider R. La procalcitonine circule chez les sujets normaux. Annales Endocrinologie 1996; suppl. 1:59.

19. Becker KL, O'Neill WJ, Snider R, Nylen E, Moore CF, Jeng J, et al. Hyperprocalcitoninemia in inhalation burn injury: a response of the pulmonary neuroendocrine cell? Anat Rec 1993; 236:136-138.

20. Becker KL, Snider R, Silva OL, Moore CF. Calcitonin heterogenity in lung cancer and medullary thyroid cancer. Acta Endocrinol 1978; 89:89-99.

21. Benador N, Siegrist CA, Gendrel D, Greder C, Benador D, Assicot M, et al. Procalcitonin is a marker of severity of renal lesions in pyelonephritis. Pediatrics 1998; 102:1422-1425.

22. Bensousan TA, Vincent F, Assicot M, Morin JF, Leclerq B, Escudier B, et al. Monokines, procalcitonin (ProCT) and opioid peptides course during a model of SIRS. Shock 1997; 8, suppl.47-48.

23. Bernard AR, Huber MB, Birnbaum RS, Aron DC, Lindall AW, Lips K, et al. Medullary thyroid carcinomas secrete a noncalcitonin peptide corresponding to the carboxyl-terminal region of preprocalcitonin. J Clin Endocrinol Metab 1983; 56:802-807.

24. Bertagna XY, Nicholson WE, Pettengill OS, Sorenson GD, Mount CD, Orth DN. Ectopic production of high molecular weight calcitonin and corticotropin by human small cell carcinoma cells in tissue culture:evidence for seperate precursors. J Clin Endocrinol Metab 1978; 47:1390-1393.

25. Bertsch T, Richter A, Hofheinz H, Bohm C, Hartel M, Aufenanger J. Procalcitonin. A new marker for acute phase reaction in acute pancreatitis. Langenbecks Arch Chir 1997; 382:367-372.

26. Bienvenu J, Monneret G, Isaac G, Bienvenu F, Putet G, Floret G. Procalcitonin in bacterial and viral infections in premature infants and neonates. Shock 1997; suppl.1.

27. Bohuon C, Petitjean S, Assicot M. Blood Procalcitonin is a new biological marker of the human septic response. New data on the specifity. Clin Intens Care suppl. 2 1994; 5:88.

28. Bone RC. Definitions for sepsis and organ failure. Crit Care Med 1992; 19:973-976.

29. Bracq S, Machason M. Calcitonin gene expression in normal human liver. FEBS 1993; 331:14-18.

30. Brain SD, Tippins JR, Morris HR, MacIntyre K, William TJ. Potent Vasodilatator activity of calcitonin gene-related peptide in human skin. J Invest Dermatol 1986; 87:533-536.

31. Brucker A. Einfluss von Procalcitonin (PCT) auf die Stimulation von Zytokinen, cycloAMP und Eicosanoiden in ausgewählten ex-vivo und in-vitro Modellen. Dissertation, FAU Erlangen-Nürnberg 1999.

33 Brunkhorst FM, Eberhard OK, Brunkhorst R. Early identification of biliary pancreatitis with PCT. Am J Gastroenterol 1998; 93:1191-1192.

34. Brunkhorst FM, Eberhard OK, Brunkhorst R. Early identification of biliary pancreatitis with procalcitonin (letter). Am J Gastroenterol 1998; 93:1191-1192.

35. Brunkhorst FM, Forycki ZF, Beier W, Wagner J. Early identification of biliary pancreatitis with PCT. A new inflammatory parameter. Gut 1995; 37 suppl. 2:111.

36. Brunkhorst FM, Forycki ZF, Wagner J. Procalcitonin immunoreactivity in severe human shock. Intens Care Med 1995; 21 suppl. 1:12.

37. Brunkhorst FM, Forycki ZF, Wagner J. Discrimination of infectious and non-infectious etiologies of the adult respiratory distress syndrome (ARDS) with procalcitonin immunoreactivity. Clin Intens Care 1995; 6:3.

38. Brunkhorst FM, Forycki ZF, Wagner J. Frühe Identifizierung der biliären Pankreatitis durch Procalcitonin – Immunreaktivität – vorläufige Ergebnisse. Chir Gastroenterol 1995; 11 suppl 2:47-50.

39. Brunkhorst FM, Forycki ZF, Wagner J. Lebensbedrohliches Glottisödem und pulmonales Hyperpermieabilitätsödem (ARDS) nach Enalapril-Exposition. Differentialdiagnostische Bedeutung der Procalcitonin-Immunreaktivität. Intensivmedizin und Notfallmedizin 1995; 32:493.

40. Brunkhorst FM, Heinz U, Forycki ZF. Kinetics of procalcitonin in iatrogenic sepsis. Intens Care Med 1998; 24:888-892.

41. Brunkhorst FM, Forycki ZF, Wagner J. Identification of immunactivation of infectious origin by procalcitonin-immunoreactivity in different body fluids. Clin Intens Care (Abstract) 1997; 7:41.

42. Camas P, Leddoux D, Vrinats Y, de Groote D, Franchimont P, Lamy M. Cytokine serum level during severe sepsis in human. Il-6 as a marker of severity. Ann Surg 1992; 215:356-362.

43. Carsin H, Assicot M, Feger F, Roy O, Pennacino I, Le Bever H, et al. Evolution and significance of circulating procalcitonin levels compared with IL-6, TNFa and endotoxin levels early after thermal injury. Burns 1997; 23:218-224.

44. Castillo MJ, Scheen AJ, Lefebvre PJ. Amylin/islet amyloid polypeptide: Biochemistry, physiology, patho-physiology. Diabet Metab 1995; 21:3-25.

45. Chiesa C, Panero A, Rossi N, Stegagno M, De Giusti M, Osborn JF, et al. Reliability of procalcitonin concentrations for the diagnosis of sepsis in critically ill neonates. Clin Infec Dis 1998; 26:664-672.

46. Dandona P, Nix D, Wilson MF, Aljada A, Love J, Assicot M, *et al.* Procalcitonin increase after endotoxin injection in normal subjects. J Clin Endocrinol Metab 1994; 79:1605-1608.

47. Davis TME, Assicot M, Bohuon C, St.John A, Li GQ, Ahn TK. Serum Procalcitonin concentrations in acute malaria. Trans R Soc Trop Med Hyg 1994; 88:670-671.

48. Davis TME, Li GQ, Sponcor JL, St.John A. Serum ionized calcium, serum and intracellular phospate, and serum parathormone concentrations in acute malaria. Trans R Soc Trop Med Hyg 1993; 87:49-53.

49. de Werra I, Jaccard C, Corradin SB, Chiolero R, Yersin B, Gallati H, *et al.* Cytokines, nitrite/nitrate, soluble tumor necrosis factor receptors, and procalcitonin concentratins: Comparisons in patients with septic shock, cardiogenic shock, and bacterial pneumonia. Crit Care Med 1997; 25:607-613.

50. Eberhard OK, Haubitz M, Brunkhorst FM, Kliem V, Koch KM, Brunkhorst R. Usefulness of procalcitonin for differentiation between activity of systemic autoimmune disease (systemic lupus erythematosus/systemic antineutrophil cytoplasmatic antibody-associated vasculitis) and invasive bacterial infection. Arthritis Rheum 1997; 40:1250-1256.

51. Eberhard OK, Haubitz M, Brunkhorst FM, Kliem V, Koch KM, Brunkhorst R. Usefulness of procalcitonin for differentiation between activity of systemic autoimmune disease (systemic lupus erythematosus/systemic antineutrophil cytoplasmic antibody-associated vasculitits) and invasive bacterial infection. Arthritis Rheum (Abstract) 1997; 40:1250-1256.

52. Eberhard OK, Langefeld I, Kuse E, Brunkhorst FM, Kliem V, Schlitt HJ, *et al.* Procalcitonin in the early phase after renal transplantation – will it add to diagnostic accuracy? Clin Transplant 1998; 12:206-211.

53. Engelmann L, Gundelach K, Pilz U, Werner M. Procalcitoinin (PCT) and its relationship to endotoxin (ETX) in sepsis. Intens Care Med 1996; 22, suppl.3:333.

54. Fabel H, Schulz A. Parameter zur Diagnose und Verlaufsbeurteilung von Infektionen in der Intensivmedizin. Intensivmed 1997; 34:466-471.

55. Findlay DM, Martin TJ. Receptors of calciotropic hormones. Horm Metab Res 1997; 29:128-134.

56. Fleischhack G, Cipic D, Juettner J, Hasan C, Bode U. Procalcitonin - a sensitive inflammation marker of febrile episodes in neutropenic children with cancer. Intens Care Med 2000; suppl. 2:202-211.

57. Fleischhack G, Cipic D, Kambeck I, Ngampolo D, Hasan C, Bode U. Procalcitonin - A sensitive marker of severe infections in neutropenic patients. (Abstract) 3rd Int Symp on Febrile Neutropenia Brussels, Dec 10-13, 1997.

58. Foce T, Bonventre JV, Flannery MR, Gorn AH, Yamin M, Goldring SR. A cloned procine renal calcitonin receptor couples to adenylyl cyclase and phospholipase C. Calcitonin Receptor Signal Transduction 1992; 1:F1110-F1115.

59. Gardinali M, Padalino P, Suffredini A, Martich GD, Hoffmann A, *et al.* Complement activation and polymorphonuclear neutrophil leukocyte elastase in sepsis. Arc Surg 1992; 127:1219-1224.

60. Gendrel D, Assicot M, Raymond J, Moulin F, Francoul C, Badoual J, et al. Procalcitonin as a marker for the early diagnosis of neonatal infection. J Pediatrics 1996; 128:570-573.

61. Gendrel D, Raymond J, Assicot M, Moulin F, Iniguez JL, Lebon P, et al. Measurement of procalcitonin levels in children with bacterial and viral meningitis. Clin Infect Dis 1997; 24:1240-1242.

62. Gendrel D, Raymond J, Assicot M, Moulin F, Lacombe C, Bergeret M, et al. Procalcitonin, IL-6 and C-reactive protein in children with severe bacterial or viral infection. 15th annual meeting of the ESPID (Abstract) 1997.

63. Gerard Y, Hober D, Assicot M, Alfandari S, Ajana F, Bourez JM, et al. Procalcitonin as a marker of bacterial sepsis in patients infected with HIV-1. J Infect 1997; 35:41-46.

64. Gerard Y, Hober D, Petitjean S, Assicot M, Bohuon C, Mouton Y, et al. High serum procalcitonin level in a 4-year old liver transplant recipient with disseminated candidiasis. Infection (letter) 1995; 23:310-311.

67. Gramm HJ, Beier W, Zimmermann J, Oedra N, Hannemann L, Boese-Landgraf J. Procalcitonin (ProCT) - A biological marker of the inflammatory response with prognostic properties. Clin Intens Care 1995; 6 suppl. 2:71.

68. Gramm HJ, Dollinger P, Beier W. Procalcitonin - ein neuer Marker der inflammatorischen Wirtsantwort. Longitudinalstudien bei Patienten mit Sepsis und Peritonitis. Chir Gastroenterol 1995; 11, suppl. 2:51-54.

69. Gramm HJ, Hannemann L. Acitivity markers for the inflammatory host response and early criteria of sepsis. Clin Intens Care 1996; 7, suppl.1:1-3.

70. Hack CE, De Groote ER, Felt-Bersma RJF, et al. Increased plasma levels of interleukin-6 in sepsis. Blood 1989; 74:1704-1710.

71. Ham J, Ellison ML, Lymoden J. Tumor calcitonin. Interaction with specific calcitonin receptors. Biochem J 1980; 190:545-550.

72. Hammer C, Staehler M, Reichart B, Schildberg FW. Differentialdiagnostik der akuten Abstossungsreaktion von Infektionen mit Procalcitonin und Zytokinen. Acta Chirurgica Austria 1997; suppl. 1:334.

73. Hammer S, Meisner F, Dirschedl P, Höbel G, Fraunberger P, Meiser B, Reichardt B, Hammer C. Procalcitonin: a new marker for diagnosis of acute rejection and bacterial infection in patients after heart and lung transplantation. Transplant Immunology 1998; 6:235-241.

74. Hammer S, Meisner F, Fraunberger P, Meiser B, Stangl M, Hammer C. Procalcitonin - Differentialdiagnose von Abstossungsreaktionen und nicht-viralen Infektionen bei Transplantationspatienten. Tx Med 1999; II:54-58

75. Hatherill M, Jones G, Lim E, Tibby M, Murdoch IA. Procalcitonin aids diagnosis of adrenocortical failure. Lancet 1997; 350:1749-1750.

76. Hensel M, Volk T, Döcke WD, Kern F, Tschirna D, Egerer K, et al. Hyperprocalcitoninemia in patients with noninfectious SIRS and pulmonary dysfunction associated with cardiopulmonary bypass. Anesthesiology 1998; 89:93-104.

77. Hergert M, Lestin HG, Scherkus M, Brinker K, Klett I, Stranz G, et al. Procalcitonin in patients with sepsis and polytrauma. Clin Lab 1998; 44:659-670.

78. Hollenstein U, Looareesuwan S, Aichelburg A, Thalhammer F, Stoiser B, Amradee S, et al. Serum procalcitonin levels in severe Plasmodium falciparum malaria. Am J Trop Med Hyg 1998; 59:860-863.

79. Huber W, Schweigart U, Bottermann P. Failure of PCT to indicate severe fungal infection in two immunodeficient patients. Infection 1997; 25:377-378.

80. Jacobs JW, Lund PK, Potts JT, Bell NH, Habener JF. Procalcitonin is a glycoprotein. J Biol Chem 1981; 256:2803-2807.

81. Janoff A. Elastase in tissue injury. Ann Rev Med 1985; 36:207-216.

82. Joyce CD. CGRP levels are elevated in patients with sepsis. Surgery 1990; (108)1097-1101.

83. Kern F, Döcke WD, Kern H, Reinke P, Jacobi C, Falke K, et al. Correlation of procalcitonin with standard immunologic parameters in ICU-patients. Shock (Abstract) 1997; 7:64.

84. Kilger E, Pichler B, Goetz AE, Rank N, Welte M, Morstedt K, et al. Procalcitonin as a marker of systemic inflammation after conventional or minimal invasive coronary artery bypass grafting. Thorac Cardiovasc Surg 1998; 46:130-133.

85. Kormos RL, Murali S, Dew MA, Aritage JM, Hardesty RL, Borovetz HS, et al. Chronic mechanical circulatory support: rehabilitation, low morbidity, and superior survival. Ann Thorac Surg 1994; 57:51-57.

86. Kou E, Giamarellos-Bourboulis J, Petrikkou E, Petrikkos G, Giamarellou H. Plasma procalcitonin (PCT) as a parameter of infection in febrile neutropenic patients. Abstract on the ICAAC, Ontario, 1997.

87. Kuhn P, Donato L, Coumaros G, Jernite M, Messer J. Interleukin-6 (Il-6) and procalcitonin (PCT) as markers for the early diagnosis of neonatal bacterial infection. 15th anual meeting of ESPID (Abstract) 1997.

88. Kuse ER, Langefeld I, Jaeger K, Külpmann WR. Procalcitonin - a new diagnostic tool in complications following liver transplantation. Intens Care Med 2000; suppl. 2:187-192.

89. Langefeld I, Schulzeck P, Schlitt HJ, Oldhafer K, Jaeger K, Kuse E-R. Procalcitonin (PCT) zur Differenzierung zwischen Infektion und Abstossung beim Transplantierten mit FUO. AINS 1997; 32:10.7.

90. Lapillonne A, Basson E, Tourneur F, Monneret G, Isaac C, Picaud JC, et al. Procalcitonin (PCT) in diagnosis of bacterial infections in newborns. 15th annual meeting of ESPID (Abstract), 1997.

91. Le Moullec JM, Jullienne A, Chenais J, Lasmoles F, Guliana JM, Milhaud G, et al. The complete sequence of human preprocalcitonin. FEBS 1984; 167:93-97.

92. Leon A, Lepouse C, Cousson J, Raclot P, Suinat JL, Assicot M, et al. Procalcitonin concentrations in pleural effusion as a marker of human septic response. Shock, suppl. (Abstract) 1995.

93. Lestin F, Lestin HG, Burstein O, Anders O, Freund M. Vorläufige Erfahrungen mit Procalcitonin, C-reaktivem Protein, Neopterin, ausgewählten Zytokinen und Hämostaseparametern an Patienten mit malignen hämatologischen Erkrankungen, bei zytostatikainduzierter Neutropenie und Fieber. Hämostase und Entzündung. Hrsg O Anders, J Jacob Weller-Verlag, Neckargemünd, 1998 1998; 1:40-52.

94. Lietzmann A. Untersuchungen zum Syntheseort und zur Induktion des neuen Infektionsparameters Procalcitonin. Dissertation, FAU-Erlangen-Nürnberg 1999.

96. Lowry SF, Calvano SE, van der Poll T. Measurements of inflammatory mediators in clinical sepsis. In: Sibbald WJ, Vincent JL (eds) Clinical trials for the treatment of sepsis. Springer, Berlin Heidelberg 1995; 1:86-105.

97. Marnitz R, Zimmermann J, Gramm H-J. Plasma procalcitonin elevation is part of the inflammatory response to major surgery. Shock (Abstract) 1997; 7:124.

98. Marty C, Misset B, Tamion F, Fitting C, Carlet J, Cavaillon JM. Circulating interleukin-8 concentrations in patients with multiple organ failure of septic and nonseptic origin. Crit Care Med 1994; 22:673-679.

99. Marx SJ, Aurbach GD, Gavin JR, Buell DW. Calcitonin receptors on cultured human lymphocytes. J Biol Chem 1974; 249:6812-6816.

100. Meisner M, Hutzler A, Tschaikowsky K, Harig F, von der Emde J. Postoperative plasma concentration of procalcitonin and C-reactive protein in patients undergoing cardiac and thoracic surgery with and without cardiopulmonary bypass. Cardiovasc Engineering 1998; 3:174-178.

101. Meisner M, Schmidt J, Huettner H, Tschaikowsky K. The natural elimination rate of procalcitonin in patients with normal and impaired renal function. Intens Care Med 2000; 26, suppl. 2:212-216.

102. Meisner M, Tschaikowsky K, Beier W, Schüttler J. Procalcitonin (PCT) - ein neuer Parameter zur Diagnose und Verlaufskontrolle von bakteriellen Entzündungen und Sepsis. Anästhesiologie und Intensivmedizin 1996; 10 (37):529-539.

103. Meisner M, Tschaikowsky K, Hutzler A, Schick C, Schüttler J. Postoperative plasma concentrations of procalcitonin after different types of surgery. Intens Care Med 1998; 24:680-684.

104. Meisner M, Tschaikowsky K, Hutzler A, Schmidt J, Harig F, von der Emde J. Postoperative plasma concentrations of procalcitonin and C-reactive protein after cardiothoracic surgery with and without extracorporeal circulation. Brit J Anaesth 1998; 80, suppl. 1:79.

105. Meisner M, Tschaikowsky K, Palmaers T, Schmidt J. Comparison of procalcitonin (PCT) and C-reactive protein (CRP) plasma concentrations at different SOFA scores during the course of sepsis and MODS. Critical Care 1999; 3:45-55.

106. Meisner M, Tschaikowsky K, Palmaers T, Schmidt J, Mangold G, Schüttler J. Comparison of procalcitonin (PCT) and C-reactive protein (CRP) plasma concentrations at different APACHE II scores during the course of sepsis and MODS. Anaesthesiology (Abstract) 1997; 87:243.

107. Meisner M, Tschaikowsky K, Palmaers T, Spegel K. Procalcitonin (PCT) and CRP: Comparison of plasma concentrations at different SOFA-scores during the course of sepsis and MODS. Shock (Abstract) 1997; 8:47.

108. Meisner M, Tschaikowsky K, Palmaers T, Spegel K, Schüttler J. Prognostische Bedeutung von Procalcitonin (PCT) bei Patienten mit Sepsis und systemischer Inflammation. Anaesthesiol Intensivmed Notfallmed Schmerzther (Abstract) 1997; 32:177.

109. Meisner M, Tschaikowsky K, Palmers T, Prudlo U, Höfig J, Schüttler J. Procalcitonin und CRP bei Sepsis und Multiorganversagen: Korrelation zu APACHE II und SOFA-Score ? Anästhesist (Abstract) 1996; 45 suppl 2:170.

110. Meisner M, Tschaikowsky K, Schmidt J, Schüttler J. Procalcitonin (PCT) - Indications for a new diagnostic parameter of severe bacterial infection and sepsis in transplantation, immunosuppression and cardiac assist devices. Cardiovasc Engineering 1996; 1:1-10.

111. Meisner M, Tschaikowsky K, Schnabel S, Schmidt J, Katalinic A, Schüttler J. Procalcitonin - Influence of temperature, storage, anticoagulation and arterial or venous asservation of blood samples on procalcitonin concentrations. Eur J Clin Chem Clin Biochem 1997; 35(8):597-601.

112. Meisner M, Tschaikowsky K, Spiessl C, Schüttler J. Procalcitonin - a marker or modulator of the acute immune response ? Intens Care Med 1996; 22 suppl 1:14.

113. Mimoz O, Benoist JF, Edouard AR, Assicot M, Bohuon C, Samii K. Procalcitonin and C-reactive protein during the early posttraumatic systemic inflammatory response syndrome. Intens Care Med 1998; 24:185-188.

114. Monneret G, Labaune JM, Isaac C, Bienvenu F, Putet G, Bienvenu J. Procalcitonin and C-reactive protein levels in neonatal infections. Acta Paediatr 1997; 86:209-212.

115. Moosig F, Csernok E, Reinhold-Keller E, Schmitt W, Gross WL. Elevated procalcitonin levels in active Wegeners granulomatosis. J Rheumatol 1998; 25:1531-1533.

116. Murray JF, Matthay MA, Luce JM, Flick MR. An expanded definition of the adult respiratory distress syndrome. Am Rev Respir Dis 1998; 138:720-723.

117. Nevalainen TJ. Serum phospholipases A2 in inflammatory diseases. Clin Chem 1993; 39:2453-2459.

118. Nylen E, Jeng J, Jordan MH, Snider R, Thompson K, Lewis MS, et al. Late pulmonary sequela following burns:persistence of hyperprocalcitoninemia using a 1-57 amino acid N-terminal flanking peptide assay. Respir Med 1995; 89:41-46.

119. Nylen E, O'Neill WJ, Jordan MH, Snider R, Moore CF, Lewis MS, et al. Serum Procalcitonin as an index of inhalation injury in burns. Horm Metab Res 1992; 24:439-442.

120. Nylen E, Snider R, Thompson KA, Rohatgi P, Becker KL. Pneumonitis-associated hyperprocalcitoninemia. Am J Med Sci 1996; 312:12-18.

121. Nylen ES, Linnoila RI, Snider RH, Tabassina AR. Comparative studies of hamster calcitonin from pulmonary endocrine cell in vitro. Peptides 1987; 8:972-982.

122. Nylen ES, Snider RH, Keith A, Thompson BS, Rohatgi P, Becker KL. Pneumonitis-associated hyperprocalcitoninemia. Am J Med Sci 1996; 312:12-18.

123. Nylen ES, Whang KT, Snider RH, Steinwald PM, White JC, Becker KL. Mortality is increased by procalcitonin and decreased by an antiserum reactive to procalcitonin in experimental sepsis. Crit Care Med 1998; 26:(6)1001-1006.

124. O'Neill WJ, Jordan MH, Lewis MS, Snider R, Moore CF, Becker KL. Serum calcitonin may be a marker for inhalation injury in burns. J Burn Care Rehabil 1992; 13:605-616.

125. Oberhoffer M, Bitterlich A, Hentschel T, Meier-Hellmann A, Vogelsang H, Reinhart K. Procalcitonin (ProCT) correlates better with the ACCP/SCCM consensus conference definitions than other specific markers of the inflammatory response. Clin Intens Care 1996; 7, suppl.1:46.

126. Oberhoffer M, Bögel D, Meier-Hellmann A, Vogelsang H, Reinhart K. Procalcitonin is higher in non-survivors during the clinical course of sepsis, severe sepsis and septic shock. Intens Care Med (Abstract) 1996; 22:A245.

127. Oberhoffer M, Karzai W, Meier-Hellmann A, Bogel D, Fassbinder J, Reinhart K. Sensitivity and specificity of various markers of inflammation for the prediction of TNF-α and IL-6 in patients with sepsis. Crit Care Med 1999; 27(9):1814-1818.

128. Oberhoffer M, Karzai W, Meier-Hellmann A, Reinhart K. Procalcitonin - ein neuer Indikator der systemischen Reaktion auf schwere Infektionen. Anaesthesist 1998; 47: 581-587.

129. Oberhoffer M, Stonans I, Russwurm S, Stonane E, Vogelsang H, Junker U, Jäger L, Reinhart K. Procalcitonin expression in human peripheral blood mononuclear cells and its modulation by lipopolysaccharides and sepsis related cytokines in vitro. J Lab Clin Med 1999; 134:49-55.

130. Oberhoffer M, Vogelsang H, Jäger L, Reinhart K. Katacalcin and calcitonin immunoreactivity in different types of leukocytes indicates intracellular procalcitonin content. J Crit Care 1999; 14:29-33.

131. Oberhoffer M, Vogelsang H, Russwurm S, Hartung T, Reinhart K. Outcome predicition by traditional and new markers of inflammation in patients with sepsis. Clin Chem Lab Med 1999; 37(3):363-368.

132. Oezcueruemez-Porsch M, Kunz D, Hardt PD, Fadgyas T, Kress O, Schulz HU, et al. Diagnostic relevance of interleukin pattern, acute-phase proteins, and procalcitonin in early phase of post-ERCP pancreatitis. Dig Dis Sci 1998; 43:1763-1769.

133. Pacher R, Redl H, Fraas M, Petzl DH, Schuster E, Woloszczuk W. Relationship between neopterin and granulocyte elastase plasma levels and the severity of multiple organ failure. Crit Care Med 1989; 17:221-226.

134. Pahlke K, Oberhoffer M, Karzai W, Meier-Hellmann A, Reinhart K. Procalcitonin – Eigenschaften eines neuen Parameters bei schweren bakteriellen Infektionen und Sepsis. Intensivmed 1997; 34:381-387.

135. Pannen B, Robotham J, Teppo A. The acute phase response. New Horiz 1995; 3:183-197.

136. Petitjean S, Assicot M. Etude de l'immunoreactivite calcitonine-like au cours des processus infectieux. Diplome d'etudes approfondies de biotechnologie, 1993; Université Paris V:1-29.

137. Petitjean S, Mackensen A, Engelhardt R, Bohuon C. Induction de la procalcitonine circulante après administration intraveneuse d'endotoxine chez l'homme. Act Pharm Biol Clin 1994; 265-268.

138. Pruzanski W, Wilmore DW, Sufredini A, Martich GD, Hoffmann AG, et al. Hyperphospholipasemia A2 in human volunteers challenged with intravenous endotoxin. Inflammation 1992; 19:561-570.

139. Rangel-Frausto MS, Pittet D, Costigan M, Hwang T, Davis C, Wenzel RP. The natural history of the systemic inflammatory response syndrome (SIRS). JAMA 1995; 273:117-123.

140. Rau B, Steinbach G, Baumgart K, Gansauge F, Grünert A, Beger HG. The clinical value of procalcitonin in the prediction of infected necrosis in acute pancreatitis. Intens Care Med 2000; 26, suppl: 2:159-164.

141. Rau B, Steinbach G, Gansauge F, Mayer M, Grünert A, Beger HG. The role of procalcitonin and interleukin-8 in the prediction of infected necrosis in acute pancreatitis. Gut 1997; 41:832-840.

142. Reinhart K. Procalcitonin: A new marker of severe infections and sepsis. Intensive care capita selecta, Ed J Bakker, Utrecht 1997; ISBN 90-72651-13-8:343-349.

143. Reinhart K, Wiegand-Lohnert C, Grimminger F, Kaul M, Withington S, Treacher D, et al. Assessment of the safety and efficacy of the monoclonal anti-tumor necrosis factor antibody-fragment, MAK 195F, in patients with sepsis and septic shock: a multicenter, randomized, placebo-controlled, dose-ranging study. Crit Care Med 1996; 24:733-742.

144. Reith HB, Lehmkuhl P, Beier W, Högby B. Procalcitonin - ein prognostischer Infektionsparameter bei der Peritonitis. Chir Gastroenterol 1995; 11 suppl 2:47-50.

145. Reith HB, Mittelkötter U, Debus ES, Kussner C, Thiede A. Procalcitonin in early detection of postoperative complications. Dig Surg 1998; 15:260-265.

146. Reith HB, Mittelkötter U, Debus ES, Lang J, Thiede A. Procalcitonin (PCT) immunreactivity in critical ill patients on a surgical ICU. The Immune Consequences of Trauma, Shock and Sepsis, Edit. Monduzzi Editore, Bologna 1997; 1:673-677.

147. Reith HB, Mittelkötter U, Endter F, Thiede A. Procalcitonin (PCT) – Anwendungsmöglichkeiten in der Chirurgie. Jahrbuch der Chirurgie, Biermann-Verlag, Köln, Germany 1999.

148. Rinalta EM, Nevalainen TJ. Group II phospholipases As in sera of febrile patients with microbiologically or clinically documented infections. Clin Infect Dis 1993; 27:864-870.

149. Rosenfeld MG, Mermod JJ, Amara SG, Swanson LW, Sawchenko PE, Rivier J, *et al.* Production of a novel neuropeptide encoded by the calcitonin gene via tissue-specific RNA processing. Nature 1983; 304:129-135.

150. Schmidt J, Meisner M, Tschaikowsky K, Schüttler J. Procalcitonin moduliert die proinflammatorische Zytokinfreisetzung in vitro. Anaesthesiol Intensivmed Notfallmed Schmerzther (Abstract) 1997; 32:171.

151. Schwenger V, Sis J, Breitbart A, Andrassy K. CRP levels in autoimmune disease can be specified by measurement of procalcitonin. Infection 1998; 26:274-276.

152. Smith MD, Suputtamongkol Y, Chaowagul W, Assicot M, Bohuon C, Petitjean S, *et al.* Elevated serum procalcitonin levels in patients with melioidosis. Clin Infect Dis 1995; 20:641-645.

153. Snider RH, Nylen ES, Becker KL. Procalcitonin and its component peptides in systemic inflammation: immunochemical characterization. J Investig Med 1997; 45:552-560.

154. Snider RH, Silva OL, Moore CF, Becker KL. Immunochemical heterogeneity of calcitonin in man: effect on radio-immunoassay. Clin Chem Acta 1977; 76:1-14.

155. Staehler M, Hammer C, Meiser B, Fürst H, Reichart B, Schildberg FW. Differential diagnostic of acute rejection and infection with procalcitonin and cytokines. Langenbecks Arch Chir /Forumband 1997; 1:205-209.

156. Staehler M, Hammer C, Meiser B, Reichart B. Procalcitonin: a new marker for differential diagnosis of acute rejection and bacterial infection in heart transplantation. Transplant Proc 1997; 29:584-585.

158. Staehler M, Überfuhr P, Reichart B, Hammer C. Differentialdiagnostik der Abstossungsreaktion und Infektion bei herztransplantierten Patienten: neue Wege mit Zytokinen und Procalcitonin als Marker. Transplantationsmedizin 1997; 9:44-50.

159. Steinwald PM, Becker KL, Nylen ES, Snider RH, White JC. Hyperprocalcitonemia of e.coli sepsis in a hamster model: association with hypocalcemia and hyperphosphatemia. Abstract on the 10th Internat Congress of Endocrinology, June 1996, San Francisco, CA 1998.

160. Tabassian AR, Nylen E, Giron AE, Snider R, Cassidy MM, Becker KL. Evidence for cigarette smoke-induced calcitonin secretion from lungs of man and hamster. Life Sci 1988; 42:2323-2329.

161. Ueyama M, Maruyama I, Osame M. Marked increase in plasma interleukin-6 in burn patients. J Lab Clin Med 1992; 120:693-698.

162. Vincent JL, Moreno R, Takala J, Willats S, De Medonca A, Bruining H, *et al.* The SOFA (Sepsis-related Organ Failure Assessment) score to describe organ dysfunction/failure. Intens Care Med 1996; 22:707-710.

163. von Heimburg D, Khorram R, Stieghorst W, Bahm J, von Saldern S. Procalcitonin (PCT) als diagnostischer und prognostischer Parameter im Krankheitsverlauf des Schwerstbrandverletzten. Handchir Mikrochir Plast Chir 1996; 28:1.

164. von Heimburg D, Stieghorst W, Khorram-Sefat R, Pallua N. Procalcitonin – a sepsis parameter in severe burn injuries. Burns 1998; 24:745-750.

165. Waydhas C, Nast-Kolb D, Jochum M, Trupka A, Lenk S, Fritz H, *et al.* Inflammatory mediators, infection, sepsis, and multiple organ failure after severe trauma. Arch Surg 1992; 127:460-467.

166. Whang KT, Steinwald PM, White JC, Nylen ES, Snider RH, Simon GL, *et al.* Serum calcitonin precursors in sepsis and systemic inflammation. J Clin Endocrinol Metab 1998; 83:3296-3301.

167. Wildling E, Pusch F, Aichelburg A, Zimpfer M, Weinstabl C. Procalcitonin is elevated in patients after severe injury. Intens Care Med (Abstract) 1997; 23:S62.

168. Zaidi M, Moonga BS, Bevis PJR, Alam ASMT, Legon S, Wimalawansa S, *et al.* Expression and function of the calcitonin gene products. Vitam Horm 1991; 46:(87)164.

169. Zeni F, Viallon A, Assicot M, Tardy B, Vindimian M, Page Y, *et al.* Procalcitonin serum concentrations and severity of sepsis. Clin Intens Care suppl 2 1994; 5:89-98.

170. Zintl F, Sauer M, Fuchs D, Hermann J, Reinhart K. High serum procalcitonin (PCT) concentrations in children and adults after hemopoietic stemm cell transplantation(HSCT) - an indicator for poor prognosis in severe infections. Blood, 1996; 88 suppl. 1:266.

171. Russwurm S, Wiederholt M, Oberhoffer M, Stonans I, Peiker G, Reinhart K. Procalcitonin als monozytärer Marker für die Frühdiagnostik bei septischem Abort. Z Geburtsh Neonatol 1999; 203:1-4.

172. Meisner M, Lohs T, Hüttemann E, Schmidt J, Reinhart K. The plasma elimination rate and urinary secretion of PCT in patients with normal and impaired renal function. Anesthesiology 1999; 91 Suppl. 3A:A236.

173. Meisner M, Lohs T, Hüttemann E, Reinhart K. Elimination of procalcitonin and plasma levels during continuous veno-venous hemofiltration in patients with acute renal failure and sepsis. Intens Care Med 1999; 25 Suppl. 15:76.

174. Meisner M, Lohs T, Hüttemann E, Reinhart K. Elimination of procalcitonin during continuous veno-venous hemodiafiltration in patients with acute renal failure and sepsis. Shock 1999; 12 Suppl.:34.

175. Meisner M. Procalcitonin: Erfahrungen mit einer neuen Meßgröße für bakterielle Infektionen und systemische Inflammation. J Lab Med 1999; 23 (5): 263-272.

176. Meisner M, Rauschmayer C, Schmidt J. Procalcitonin indicates increased risk after cardiovascular surgery. Shock 1999; 12 Suppl.:16-17.

177. Hoffmann G, Seibel M, Smolny M, Schobersberger W: Procalcitonin suppresses inducible nitric oxide synthase in vascular smooth muscle cells. Intens Care Med 1999; 25 Suppl. 1:75.

178. Meisner M, Rotgeri A, Brunkhorst FM. Ein semiquantitativer Schnelltest zur Bestimmung von Procalcitonin. J Lab Med 2000; 24(2):76-85.

179. Nylen E, Muller B, Snider R, Vath S, Wagner K, White J, Zulewsk H, Vannier E, Habener J, Becker K. Pathophysiological significance of calcitonin precursors in sepsis and systemic inflammation. Shock 1999; 12 Suppl.:14.

180. Whang KT, Vath SD, Nylen ES, Muller B, Qichang Li, Tamarkin L, White JC. Procalcitonin and proinflammatory cytokine interactions in sepsis. Shock 1999; 12(4):265-273.

181. Brunkhorst FM, Clark AL, Forycki ZF, Anker SD. Pyrexia, procalcitonin, immune activation and survival in cardiogenic shock: the potential importance of bacterial translocation. Int J Card 1999; 72: 3-10.

182. Wrenger S, Kahne T, Bohuon C, Weglöhner W, Ansorge S, Reinhold D. Aminoterminal truncation of procalcitonin, a marker for systemic bacterial infections, by dipeptidyl peptidase IV CDP IV. FEBS Lett 2000, 466(1): 155-159.

183. Kuse ER, Langefeld I, Jaeger K, Kulpmann WR. Procalcitonin in fever of unknown origin after liver transplantation: a variable to differentiate acute rejection from infection. Crit Care Med 2000; 28(2):555-9.